CHILD OBESITY

CHILD OBESITY

A
Parent's
Guide to a Fit,
Trim, and Happy Child

GOUTHAM RAO, MD

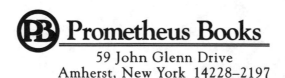

Prometheus Books

59 John Glenn Drive
Amherst, New York 14228–2197

*62282277

Published 2006 by Prometheus Books

Inquiries should be addressed to
Prometheus Books
59 John Glenn Drive
Amherst, New York 14228–2197
VOICE: 716–691–0133, ext. 207
FAX: 716–564–2711
WWW.PROMETHEUSBOOKS.COM

10 09 08 07 06   5 4 3 2 1

Library of Congress Cataloging-in-Publication Data

Rao, Goutham.
Child obesity : a parent's guide to a fit, trim, and happy child / Goutham Rao.
p. cm.
Includes bibliographical references and index.
ISBN 1-59102-377-7 (pbk. : alk. paper) 1. Obesity in children—United States—Popular works. 2. Obesity in children—United States—Prevention—Popular works.
I. Title.
RJ399.C6R36 2006
618.92'398--dc22

2005032628

Printed in the United States of America on acid-free paper

Contents

Preface   7

Introduction   11

Chapter One How Bad Is the Problem?   24

Chapter Two "Liquid Candy":
              Kids Raised on Soft Drinks   44

Chapter Three Fast-Food Epidemic   57

Chapter Four Mesmerized by the Screen: Television
              and Other Media   68

Chapter Five Bodies Not in Motion: Physical Activity
              and Its Role in Weight Control   84

Chapter Six The Family Meal in the Twenty-first Century   101

Chapter Seven The Truth about Diets, Programs,
            and Other Products   115

Chapter Eight The Science of Changing Behavior
            and Its Role in Weight Control   131

Chapter Nine A Rational Approach to Achieving or
            Maintaining a Healthy Weight   145

Chapter Ten Advocacy for a Healthier "Built Environment"   167

Chapter Eleven A Glimpse of the Future   185

Chapter Twelve Stories of Three Children   200

Afterword   211

Notes   215

Web Resources   239

Index   241

Preface

I first came to Pittsburgh in 1996 to begin a job as a family physician and member of the faculty of a family medicine training program. Among my responsibilities was working aboard a community health van that provided care to residents of housing projects and other underprivileged communities in the city. The van was actually a doctor's office on wheels. It was immense—as big as the largest RVs sold today. It was so heavy that all its tires needed to be replaced every four thousand miles. Inside were two exam rooms, a refrigerator for vaccines, a telephone, a radio, and plenty of other medical supplies. I first met Tawanda Harris (not her real name) in 1997. She was a pretty, tall, slim, shy fifteen-year-old African American girl who attended high school and worked part-time at a fast-food outlet. She came aboard the van to discuss her acne. I gave her some advice together with a prescription for retinoic acid cream for her face and asked her to call my office to arrange a follow-up appointment. My office was quite far away from where she and her mother lived, so I told her another option would be to return to the van in a couple of weeks or to find a doctor near her home.

I didn't see Tawanda again until two years later. She was still in high school but had found a different part-time job in the inner-city neighborhood in which my practice is located. She was registering at the front desk as a new patient when she saw me behind the receptionist. "Dr. Rao. How've you been?"

I replied reflexively, "I've been well and you?" At first I really didn't recognize her. No wonder. Tawanda was 5'10" tall and stepped on our office scale that day at 247 lbs.—more than 100 lbs. heavier than she had been just two years earlier. She came to see me to discuss her weight and what she could do about it. I wasn't sure how and where to begin. The transformation was incredible. She didn't look like a seventeen-year-old girl. Tawanda's face had the same features but seemed "puffed up." She wore a T-shirt and huge, ugly cotton sweatpants that her legs filled up completely. She looked like a forty-year-old woman who had had a hard life. My first question to her was, "How did this happen?"

Tawanda's case isn't unusual and is the final product of the complex interplay of a number of factors: unhealthy food in her environment; complete lack of exercise; failure to realize initially the consequences of being overweight or obese; and a mother (herself overweight) who didn't think Tawanda's weight was a problem. The purpose of this book is to help you understand how a few specific culprits have contributed so much to the epidemic of obesity now destroying the health of American children. The book will let you know how to help not only your child, whose health is of the utmost importance to you, but also how you can contribute to improving the health of all children. Included are stories of children and their parents who fought and won battles against overweight and obesity. Their successes were based upon careful attention to good eating habits, regular exercise, and the cultivation at an early age of a range of other behaviors that are consistent with a long and healthy life.

I am astounded by how many diet books are on the market. Some of these are intended for children. You won't find any new diets in this book. You also won't find any "magic" bullets that will make your child thin overnight. I have included, however, a chapter on emerging therapies such as new drugs and surgeries that can benefit a small number of children whose weight problem is especially severe.

There is plenty of information available to the general public about how to deal with childhood weight problems. Unfortunately, much of it is simply drawn from one author's opinion or from experience with overweight and obese adults. The information in this book is based upon the latest and most sound evidence available in the scientific literature about childhood obesity. Reference lists are included for each chapter. I encourage you to read as much as you can. This book is only a start.

I am extremely grateful to the following individuals for their thoughtful reviews of this book as I wrote it. Not only did I benefit from their advice and expertise, but also from their own personal experiences both as children and parents: Michelle Bretzing, JD; Joel Merenstein, MD; Anita Rao, MD; Sukanya Srinivasan, MD, MPH; Henry Willis, PhD; and Dorothy Wilson, MD.

Introduction

WHY I WROTE THIS BOOK

An interesting way for me to explain why this book is important for you and your child is to tell you why and how I came to write it. It is in everyday clinical practice that I developed an interest in and experience with childhood obesity. I'm currently the clinical director of the Weight Management and Wellness Center at Children's Hospital of Pittsburgh and associate professor of pediatrics at the University of Pittsburgh School of Medicine. I have been both a professor and practicing physician for ten years. Let me start by telling you a bit about what that's like. I think it will help you understand my perspective on this significant problem.

Primary care is a challenging field for several reasons. A patient can walk into my office with just about any problem. Over the course of a single day, I see a mix of children, young adults, families, and the elderly. The problems my patients have are remarkably varied. I'll diagnose and treat migraine, pneumonia, and middle ear infection in a single afternoon, for example.

I spend a great deal of my time teaching medical students about family medicine. One of their major concerns when they arrive at my office is that there are simply too many different problems to evaluate and treat. I often hear, "How can anyone possibly know enough about everything to take good care of patients?" To make things easier, I explain to them that though it is true that the typical primary care patient can walk into the office with any type of problem, the majority of patients will usually have one or more of a relatively short list of different problems.

Every medical specialty has its own short list. Physicians refer to this as the "bread and butter" of their discipline. To help students learn, I divide the bread and butter of primary care into three categories: looking after the most common "acute" or short-lived problems; doing checkups on patients who generally feel well; and looking after the most common chronic problems. Common acute problems include things like upper and lower respiratory tract infections, sports injuries, and headaches. What comprises a checkup for a patient depends upon the patient's age and medical and family history. Typical checkups for children, for example, include screening for lead poisoning, reminding parents to use child safety car seats, and administering immunizations.

It is the last category, the management of chronic diseases, that many physicians and other healthcare providers find the most challenging. Common chronic diseases include diabetes, high blood pressure, and asthma. Patients with these problems are seen at regular intervals. The severity of their disease is monitored and adjustments are made to medications and other treatments. It's also important to check for complications of chronic diseases. Diabetes, for example, can lead to kidney failure. Regular testing for kidney failure, therefore, is part of checkups for diabetes. The challenge in caring for patients with chronic illnesses is not in making a diagnosis. It isn't hard, for example, to figure out if a child has asthma. Caring for a patient with a chronic disease is challenging because so much of the patient's quality of life depends not on what the physician does, but on what the patient does.

A big part of the role of the physician in caring for a patient with a chronic illness is to provide information on how the patient can best look after himself or herself. Consider the following example. A sixteen-year-old boy came to me with a fractured wrist. I obtained an x-ray, diagnosed a fracture, put his wrist in a cast, asked him to take his pain medications as he needed them, stressed the importance of keeping his cast clean and dry for four weeks, and asked him to return to see me. His part of the plan is fairly simple. All he had to do was to keep his cast on and use his medication for comfort.

Another teenager came to see me for her asthma checkup. She also has seasonal allergies. I prescribed her medications for these problems a few years ago, but she often forgot or didn't feel like taking some of them. I advised her to keep a diary of her symptoms, so she could identify "triggers" that make her worse. She told me she can't find the time or doesn't feel like she has the energy or motivation to do that. Unfortunately, she recently started smoking. I advised her to quit and offered her help. She declined because she didn't think she was quite ready to take that step in her life, especially as school had recently become very stressful.

Children with asthma can check their lung function with a simple device called a peak flow meter. The child breathes out into the device as hard and as fast as possible. A low peak flow is a warning that an asthma flare is imminent. I asked my patient to check her peak flow daily. She agreed to do this but stopped doing it after awhile. She told me she can now usually "feel when she is about to get sick" and doesn't feel the need to use the peak flow meter every day. In cases such as this, I have the simple part. I check the severity of her illness and for complications. I do my best to encourage her to do the right things. I spend a big part of her visits trying to motivate her to take better care of herself. Her part of the deal is much, much bigger and harder. This is what we physicians sometimes find frustrating. There is only so much we can do about chronic illness. Patients must do the rest.

Last year the federal government, through its Medicare program, officially recognized obesity as a "disease." The medical community has recognized obesity as a common chronic illness with serious consequences for some time. Among chronic illnesses, obesity is like no other. In contrast to high blood pressure or diabetes, it isn't at all hard for anyone to identify. Often people with high blood pressure or diabetes generally feel just fine. Obese people usually know they're obese. They *feel* their disease every time they buy clothes or board a bus or an airplane. They feel pain through stigmatization and social isolation. They feel the burden of their extra weight when they climb a flight of stairs.

It is, of course, very easy to diagnose obesity. Most physicians, however, myself included, find it awfully hard to even bring up the issue of obesity or weight-related issues in general with their patients. Weight is an extremely sensitive issue for many people. I find it easier to ask an adult patient about her sexual habits than to raise the issue of weight without sounding pejorative or judgmental.

Some physicians are far too subtle in how they raise the issue. During an encounter with a middle-aged man, a medical resident I was supervising identified obesity as one of his chronic problems. He dealt with the patient's high blood pressure and his heartburn skillfully. At the end of the encounter, looking both embarrassed and a little nervous, he said, "Well, your weight today is 245 pounds. That's up three pounds from the last visit." He waited anxiously for the patient to respond in some way. He didn't. The resident continued, "Well, that's it for today's visit unless you have any questions." The patient had none. As timid as his approach may seem, at least the resident mentioned the patient's weight. Surveys have shown that many physicians consciously avoid discussing weight altogether

I've tried a number of different approaches to raising the issue of weight, some more successful than others. "Sneaking in" the issue with patients, in my experience, is not a good idea. A few years ago, a teenager came to me seeking treatment for stress and anxiety, which she attributed to an unstable relationship with her family. She was very obese. Since she hadn't seen a doctor in some time, I provided a complete checkup together with some tips on how to deal with stress. During this discussion, I sneaked in, "You know, exercise is definitely a good way to relieve stress for many people. Even simple exercise like walking. It would also help you lose weight which is also important." The patient's face turned a little red. She immediately became quiet and withdrawn. She seemed cold, angry, and offended for the rest of the encounter. I learned a valuable lesson.

I believe the best way for physicians and all other healthcare professionals to raise the issue of weight with their patients is to be nonjudgmental but perfectly direct, something to this effect: "You're weight today is 235 pounds. That makes you 65 pounds overweight. This is a serious problem that we need to discuss." More healthcare professionals need to do this. Some people will always be offended by this approach. A couple of years ago, a school district in Pennsylvania became the first to send children home not only with report cards but also with a report on their weight, including whether they were overweight or obese. Hundreds of parents were offended and furious. Hundreds of others were not and found the information helpful.

There may always be some stigma associated with being overweight or obese and that may hinder physicians from dealing with the problem effectively. I'm optimistic that this will improve over the course of time. Consider depression and other mental illnesses. Depression is now recognized as a serious chronic illness that affects the way people work, learn, and interact with others. It takes a tremendous toll on our society in general. Twenty years ago, patients with depression were embarrassed if not ashamed of their diagnosis. Today television commercials feature attractive people overcoming depression with the help of medication. I even hear people in public comparing their responses to different medications for depression. Patients don't hesitate to tell me that they're depressed.

Depression is out of the closet. Obesity, of course, is still in the closet. Physicians and others still have an enormous amount of trouble having open and honest discussions about it. Throughout society, people are uncomfortable discussing obesity. This makes obesity especially prone to misinformation. Wait in a checkout line in a super-market and you'll see at least one tabloid newspaper promising some sort of miracle for weight loss. Late-night infomercials feature attractive, athletic models pushing uncomfortable and cheap-looking exercise equipment. Walk into a nutritional supplement store and you'll find a host of "fat burners" that promise to melt away the pounds effortlessly.

Most rational people realize that losing weight isn't that easy. Yet falling prey to misinformation and sometimes out of desperation, Americans spend billions of dollars a year on themselves and their children on largely ineffective weight-loss schemes and products. If they're getting little or no help from their physicians, people will seek help elsewhere.

Physicians find it hard to discuss weight-related issues with their patients not only because weight is a sensitive topic but also because they feel their capacity to help is so limited. The patient's role in the successful treatment of obesity is bigger than that in any other chronic disease. I do find caring for patients with diabetes frustrating, but at least I can provide a range of treatments that I know are useful in preventing and treating complications of the disease. A physician has very few weapons in his or her arsenal for the battle against obesity. There are a few medications currently available and more on the way, but for many people, their effectiveness remains questionable. Physicians can provide sensible recommendations about how to lose weight or maintain a healthy weight. Their ability to encourage or motivate patients to follow those recommendations, however, is limited.

It is hard enough for physicians to help their adult patients with weight-related issues, but it is even more challenging to help overweight and obese children for several reasons. Weight is often an even more sensitive issue among children. A colleague of mine, caring for an obese twelve-year-old boy brought in by his mother, decided to raise the issue of the boy's weight in a careful and respectful manner. He showed the mother the boy's growth chart, which indicated that the boy was well above the 95th percentile of body weight for boys of the same weight and height. He also reviewed the consequences of obesity. As he began this discussion, the boy sat quietly, but his mother got very angry and said, "Okay, let's put an end to this right now. Jason is very sensitive about these things. I can't believe you're talking about this!"

Adults are generally able to understand the medical consequences of obesity. I have had many detailed discussions with adult patients about how losing weight will help them get their blood sugar or blood pressure under control, or how it will put less stress on their joints. Most children do not have this kind of understanding. I once tried to motivate an eleven-year-old girl to watch her diet and to exercise to lose weight by telling her that if she continued with her bad habits, she might develop diabetes when she got older. I went on to explain that diabetes could cause her to go blind or to lose a limb. She looked at me skeptically and said, "Nah. . . . Eating too many chips will make you blind? I never heard that before." Children also have less ability to follow recommendations for achieving or maintaining a healthy weight than adults. I can ask an overweight or obese adult, for example, to walk for thirty minutes a day every evening as a way to promote weight loss. Many adults can incorporate an evening walk into their daily routines. It is easy for them to keep track of how far or for how long to walk. Children have more difficulty putting these kinds of recommendations into practice. A child asked to walk thirty minutes a day may have trouble making this a regular, structured habit.

I direct a center that specializes in pediatric obesity in a large children's hospital. The center has physicians, nutritionists, psychologists, researchers, exercise physiologists, and nurses—all of whom have expertise in obesity. We have the latest equipment and access to the best treatments. Even *all of us put together* can do only a relatively small part in helping a child maintain or achieve a healthy weight. Some schools have recently adopted policies to raise awareness of obesity and to promote healthy lifestyles. I believe that these policies are wise, but more is needed. Like physicians, educators are limited in their ability to tackle this important problem. Teachers are certainly not comfortable raising the issue of weight with individual students. Measures like sending home "weight report cards" help raise awareness but don't offer practical solutions for weight problems. Some schools are making more nutritional foods available and getting rid of "junk food." This is a good step forward but will have a limited effect if a child indulges in junk food at home. As a parent, you, more than anyone, can help your child achieve or maintain a healthy weight. No one else who accepts this challenge can be as supportive, motivated, or diligent. The best way for me to help is to help you to help your child. This is why I wrote this book.

WHO SHOULD READ THIS BOOK?

This book is intended for any parent, guardian, or anyone else concerned about the problem of childhood obesity. Its purpose is to promote understanding of both the causes of childhood obesity and the behaviors that are consistent with achieving or maintaining a healthy weight. You are in the best position to help your child, and in order to do so, you need the best possible information and tips on how to use it. The book is not only for those with overweight or obese children. I am confident that all parents will find it helpful.

A FRESH APPROACH: THE STORY OF EVIDENCE-BASED MEDICINE

Simple ideas that aren't necessarily based on something extraordinarily new can sometimes be revolutionary. One such idea was born in Canada in the late 1960s. A new medical school was established at McMaster University in Hamilton, Ontario. Starting a new medical school is no easy feat. In the United States only one entirely new school, Florida State University School of Medicine, has been established in the last twenty years. One of the great challenges is to establish a good reputation to attract the best students and faculty. A new school must compete with prestigious, well-established institutions, which not only enjoy great reputations but also often have enormous human and financial resources. This was the situation in which the new McMaster medical school found itself. In Canada, the medical schools of McGill University and the University of Toronto, both within a day's drive, were among the world's best. Renowned medical schools in the northeastern and midwestern United States like Harvard, the University of Michigan, and the University of Chicago dwarfed McMaster's fledgling school in status and money. All these competitive institutions were hotbeds of scientific and medical research—responsible for many discoveries that have changed the practice of medicine and the quality of life for millions of people around the world.

Instead of building a medical school in the image of established, well-respected institutions, the founders of McMaster's school decided to develop, from scratch, a fresh approach to the way medicine is both taught and practiced. The opportunity to participate in the building of a medical school based on innovation attracted distinguished faculty from across North America. McMaster quickly became a leader in innovations in medical education. A young physician from Chicago, Dr. David Sackett, was among the innovators pulled north to McMaster. Sackett is the founder of the modern discipline known as *evidence-based medicine,* often abbreviated "EBM." EBM actually traces its origins to nineteenth-century Paris. It doesn't deal with any specific part of the body, nor any specific laboratory technique or treatment. Its premise is remarkably simple: The decisions that physicians make about the care of their patients should be guided by the best available scientific literature in combination with their own experience and their patients' preferences. This certainly doesn't seem revolutionary. I think most patients believe that the care they receive from their physicians is always based on the best research studies. The reality is quite different. Some of the care patients receive is poorly grounded in science. Physicians sometimes make decisions based on what *they think* is the right thing to do based on their experience. This is not always consistent with what the scientific literature, or "evidence," shows. A patient who visits her physician for a simple or complex problem may receive care based only on the physician's opinion. The proponents of EBM don't recommend abandoning opinion and experience in the care of patients. They only ask that physicians systematically and conscientiously identify and interpret the latest scientific evidence and incorporate it into patient care.

EBM has received an increasing amount of attention in the medical community in recent years: 648 scientific articles were published about EBM in 1997; 1,845 were published in 2000; and 2,680 were published in 2003. The number of physicians and other healthcare professionals regularly using evidence to help guide decisions is also slowly and steadily increasing. Armed with articles about the latest medical research printed off the Internet (some of which unfortunately are of questionable reliability), patients themselves are asking their physicians tough questions about new diagnostic tests and treatments. EBM is actually part of a larger movement in our society toward more standardized, higher-quality care and more accountability, not only by physicians, but also by the healthcare system in general.

The care of chronic diseases, like that for any problem, should be evidence-based. This applies to both the physician's and the patient's role in treating disease. When I care for a patient with diabetes, I prescribe the optimal combination of medications to keep his blood sugar under control, because I know that the evidence shows that good control of blood sugar helps prevent complications like blindness. When I ask a patient with diabetes to take good care of his or her feet (such as not walking barefoot), I do so not because *I think* it's a good idea but because *I know* that there is strong scientific evidence that good foot care among diabetic patients is associated with fewer injuries to and nasty infections of the skin. Since patients must play a huge role in looking after their own weight problems, it makes sense that the information they use for this is also based on the best evidence. Put another way, if doctors now have access to and are encouraged to use the best evidence in caring for patients, why shouldn't patients use the same approach in caring for themselves? Unfortunately, much of the weight-related information available to patients is not evidence-based.

While doing research for this book, I went to a local bookstore in my neighborhood with the goal of counting the number of diet and nutrition books for sale and glancing through the table of contents of each one. I realized pretty soon that this was impossible. There was one entire aisle just for "low-carb" diet books. There were two other aisles featuring different approaches to weight loss. I learned later that there are more than twelve hundred diet books currently on the market including a significant number that target young children and teens. Americans spent $1.38 billion on diet books, tapes, and exercise videos in 2002 and are expected to spend $1.76 billion on the same items in 2006. I came across some bizarre diet books during my brief survey that recommend everything from eating only uncooked food to eating a limited variety of foods that have been selected to boost a child's school performance. Do these exotic diets deliver what they promise to adults and children? I have no idea. I do know that these and many other diet books are not evidence-based. No one has carefully evaluated their effectiveness and safety.

There are, however, some excellent nutrition and weight-loss books and other products on the market. These have some important characteristics. First, credible books do not make outrageous claims like "lose weight overnight!" Second, the recommendations that they make have a widely accepted biological basis. For example, it makes sense to reduce the size of portions of the foods one eats in order to lose weight since that reduces the number of calories taken in. By contrast, there is no reason to think that eating raw food causes weight loss or that one's blood type is related to the types of foods one should consume to lose weight. There is nothing in the vast body of knowledge of human physiology that is consistent with these claims. Finally, the effectiveness of different reputable diets and programs is supported by evidence. It is not enough to claim that a diet will cause a weight loss of 50 lbs. Readers should look for proof.

I have done my utmost in this book to provide evidence from the scientific literature that supports each important fact and recommendation. That's why there are so many references. The references are available should you wish to retrieve the evidence behind the facts, either because of your own doubts or simply because you'd like to read more about specific topics. For your convenience, I've used as many Internet sources as possible for references of scientific and other articles. You can read short summaries of most of the scientific article references that do not include a direct Web link by punching in the titles and authors' names in the National Library of Medicine's PubMed search engine, located at http://www.pubmed.com. I've also included some valuable additional Web resources at the end of the book.

Evidence-based books include references to the evidence, but not all books that have references are evidence-based. I've found many books promoting some pretty ludicrous diets that include extensive bibliographies. How one approaches the task of writing a book is also important. Many authors of diet books and other self-help materials begin with a preconceived notion of what they think works or what they wish to promote, and then search through the enormous number of articles ever published to find a few that support their views. This is akin to a politician who, during a recession, decides to give an upbeat speech about the economy and plucks some positive economic statistics out of what is an overall bleak picture. The way in which evidence is gathered should be systematic.

Before writing this book, I certainly had some ideas about how children can best achieve or maintain a healthy weight. My beliefs were based partly on my experience as a physician and some important articles and books I had read. I knew this wasn't good enough. I started with a clean slate, putting aside my preconceived ideas, at least temporarily. I searched electronic databases for all scientific articles published about childhood obesity over the past ten years and assessed each for scientific merit and usefulness. I also consulted experts in the field of obesity, both here in Pittsburgh and elsewhere, to incorporate their perspectives on the solution to this important and common childhood problem. This book is the product of this exhaustive, systematic approach to gathering scientific evidence combined with my own observations developed over several years in caring for obese children.

HOW THIS BOOKS IS STRUCTURED

This book is divided into two parts. My first goal is to bring to your attention the causes and severity of childhood obesity in America. This serves two purposes. First, I am hopeful that it will provide a stimulus for you to become more aware of weight problems not only among your own children but also in your own community. An army of parents, well educated about childhood obesity, can make a huge difference by becoming advocates for changes to our environment, such as including more physical education in schools, which are consistent with healthy weights and good overall health. Second, I strongly believe that an educated parent is better able to help a child make changes in his behavior to achieve or maintain a healthy weight. You are better prepared to encourage your child to cut back on junk food, for example, if you understand exactly *how* unhealthy some junk food is.

The second part of the book includes a set of recommendations designed to promote healthy weight among children. There is no magic bullet for the problem of childhood obesity and I have not invented one for this book. You will find sensible advice that may not make an overweight child thin overnight, but in the long run will help him or her become fit, trim, and happy. A glimpse of the future of obesity care and research follows these recommendations. At the end of the book you will find stories about obese children who, with the help of their parents, have successfully implemented recommendations for weight loss. These stories are composites based on actual cases I've encountered as clinical director of the Weight Management Center of Children's Hospital of Pittsburgh. I've deliberately used a broad selection of children for the stories. I am hopeful that one of these kids will resemble your own son or daughter in some ways so that this book will be especially personally meaningful to you.

Chapter One

How Bad Is the Problem?

F ive years ago, while preparing a talk on childhood obesity, I came across an Internet archive of class photos of children who had attended one tiny rural Florida elementary school between the 1930s and 1990s. The old black-and-white photographs from the 1930s and 1940s showed very thin groups of children. Some of these pictures were taken during the height of the Great Depression, and at least a few of the kids were undoubtedly moderately undernourished. Pictures from the 1950s and 1960s showed less somber, more playful children. There were one or two obviously heavyset kids in some photographs, but most were wiry. Photographs from the 1970s and early 1980s (color) were similar. Gradually through the late 1980s and 1990s, the number of overweight children in the photographs began to increase. The newest photographs showed classes in which the majority of children were overweight or obese.

Obesity, both among children and adults, has received an enormous amount of media attention in recent years. Between October 1999 and October 2000, 395 media reports about obesity (newspaper articles, TV reports, and Internet reports) were released in English and available to Americans. Between October 2002 and October 2003, this number had grown to 4,767.[1] In 2003 the American Public Health Association held a forum titled "Is Childhood Obesity the Next Tobacco?" Indeed, obesity is getting the kind of attention both among the public and the medical community in the new millennium that smoking received in the 1990s. The reason for the increased attention paid to obesity, however, is quite different. The number of smokers in America remained either steady or declined modestly over the past thirty years. In other words, smoking didn't get any worse for a long time. The importance of smoking as a public health problem increased in the 1990s because of high-profile lawsuits filed against the tobacco companies. On the other hand, childhood obesity is getting more attention because the number of obese children, as the school photographs demonstrated, is increasing at an alarming rate. The problem is quickly getting worse so society is trying desperately to react. It is spreading across America like an uncontrollable virus. No wonder the word "epidemic" often follows "childhood obesity" in the news media.

OBESITY BY THE NUMBERS

Is all the attention paid to childhood obesity justified? I do think that some media reports are unnecessarily pessimistic. I've frequently read or heard the statement, "Today's children will be the first generation ever not to outlive its parents because of obesity." The underlying assumption is that children will continue becoming more obese and the consequences will be more severe, shortening their lifespan. Only time will tell if this prediction is true. I am actually optimistic that as we all become more aware of the problem of childhood obesity, we will find sensible and effective solutions. Making long-range predictions based on the extent of today's obesity epidemic is at best imprecise and at worst creates a false sense of hopelessness about the future of America's children. That having been said, obesity is a very common problem that needs to be taken very seriously.

There are several different ways to define obesity. Obesity is an excess of body fat. Unfortunately, accurately measuring the amount of body fat a person has isn't easy and requires expensive and cumbersome equipment. The most accurate way is to weigh the person while fully submerged for a few seconds in a tank of water. This method yields an accurate measure of the body's density. Since fat is less dense than muscle or bone, the density can be used to calculate the percentage of body fat. This technique is limited to specialized facilities. You can imagine that many people aren't thrilled about being fully submerged in water. Simple measures based on height and weight, though less accurate, are much more practical. In 1942 Louis Dublin, a statistician with the Metropolitan Life Insurance Company, studied the records of four million insured customers and discovered that those who lived longest maintained a body weight equivalent to that of the average twenty-five-year-old, adjusted for sex, height, and body-frame size. Based on this observation, Dublin developed charts of "ideal weights" for men and women. These became widely accepted standards over many years for the insurance industry, healthcare professionals, and the general public.

Today the most widely accepted standard used to define obesity is based upon the *body mass index* or BMI. Like the old Metropolitan Life Insurance Tables, the BMI takes both height and weight into account. The BMI is calculated using kilograms (metric measure for weight) and meters (metric measure for height). One kilogram is 2.2 lbs. One meter is 39 inches:

BMI = weight (kg)/height (m) × height (m)

Below is a formula that uses inches and pounds with which Americans are more familiar:

BMI = [weight in pounds/height (inches) × height (inches)] × 703

Consider this example. A man weighs 165 lbs. and is 5'9" (or 69") tall. His BMI is therefore,

= [165/(69 × 69)] × 703 = 24.4

The BMI is measured in units of kilograms/meters squared. At first, this may seem like an obscure way of defining obesity. It isn't hard to say that someone who weighs 300 lbs. is obese, but what does a BMI of 30 kg/m^2 mean? The National Institutes of Health (NIH) have defined cutoff levels for adults and children that are helpful in defining the health risk associated with a particular body weight. Adults with a BMI less than 18.5 are *underweight.* Those with a BMI between 18.5 and 24.9 have a *healthy* weight. Those with a BMI between 25.0 and 29.9 are *overweight.* Obesity is defined as a BMI of 30 or more. There are also subcategories of obesity based on BMI. Adults with a BMI of 30.0 to 34.9 have *grade 1 obesity*; those with a BMI of 35 to 39.9 have *grade 2 obesity*; those with a BMI of 40 or more have *grade 3* or what is commonly known as morbid obesity. According to these cutoffs, a healthy weight for an adult who is 5'7" tall is between 118 lbs. and 160 lbs. A weight between 160 lbs. and 191 lbs. is overweight, and a weight greater than 191 lbs. is obese. The BMI does have some disadvantages. Bone and muscle are heavier than fat. The BMI does not take this into account. A very athletic and muscular individual, for example, may be classified as obese, even though the amount of body fat he has may be quite low. Similarly, though men have significantly more muscle and bone mass than women, separate cutoffs of BMI for men and women are not used. Health professionals believe, however, that the BMI's simplicity as a measure of obesity supercedes these limitations. There just aren't that many very muscular people, and though men are generally heavier than women, both men and women with a BMI of more than 25 are at significantly increased risk of serious health problems.

The BMI is also used to define obesity among children, but here the situation is a bit more complicated. Children gain weight not only as they grow taller but also as their bodies mature. Puberty is associated with significant weight gain even though height may not increase proportionately. Girls also reach puberty before boys. To account for these changes, age and sex are taken into consideration when using BMI to determine if a child is obese. According to the Centers for Disease Control (CDC),[2] if a child has a BMI that is at or greater than 85% and less than 95% of that of children of the same age and sex, he or she is *at risk for overweight.* When the BMI exceeds that of 95% of children of the same age and sex, the child is *overweight.* The term "obese" is considered by some to be pejorative. The CDC does not use it at all to describe children. "At risk for overweight" among children is equivalent, however, to "overweight" among adults, and "overweight" among children is equivalent to "obese" among adults. I believe separate terms for adults and children are confusing. To keep things simple, I use the terms "overweight" and "obese" for both adults and children throughout this book.

The best information about the number of overweight and obese adults and children comes from the National Health and Nutrition Examination Survey (NHANES), which is completed annually by the federal government. A large sample of adults and children are assessed carefully for obesity and a number of other problems. The 2002 survey, results of which are the most recent available, reveals staggering percentages of overweight and obese adults and children within this large sample:[3] 65.7% of all adults surveyed were classified as *either* overweight or obese; 30.6% of all adults surveyed were obese; 5.1% were morbidly obese. In other words, only about one-third of American adults were of a normal, healthy weight. Though less common than among adults, the percentages of overweight and obese children were extremely high: 31% of all children ages 6 through 19 surveyed were *either* overweight or obese; 16.0% were obese. Obesity is becoming common even among very young children: 10.4% of children ages 2 through 5 were obese according to a survey conducted in 1999–2000.[4]

As disturbing as the overall numbers of overweight and obese adults and children are, weight problems are even more common among certain segments of the population. Soon after I arrived in Pittsburgh, I organized a health fair in an inner-city African American neighborhood, to provide screening for obesity, diabetes, and hypertension. The majority of people who participated were young women.

The fair was held over two days. At the end of the first day, I realized I hadn't seen a single woman who *wasn't* overweight or obese. Nationwide, 77.2% of all African American women are either overweight or obese; 49.0% or nearly half are obese.[5] Obesity is also much more common among Mexican American women than among the general population. The picture among minority children is also discouraging: 35.4% of African American children 6 through 19 are either overweight or obese; 20.5% are obese. Of Mexican American children 6 through 19, 39.9% are either overweight or obese; 22.2% are obese. Mexican American boys are more likely to be overweight or obese than either white or African American boys. Like African American women, African American girls 6 through 19 are more likely than other girls the same age to be overweight (40.1% versus 30.3% of all girls) or obese (23.2% versus 15.1% of all girls).[6]

Not only are overweight and obesity common problems among American children, but there is evidence that the epidemic has accelerated dramatically in recent years.[7] Between 1963 and 1970 the percentage of children who were obese was relatively constant: 4.2% of children ages 6 through 11 were obese; 4.6% of children 12 through 19 were obese. Between 1976 and 1980 these numbers had risen modestly: 6.5% of children ages 6 through 11 were obese; 5.0% of children ages 12 through 19 were obese. More dramatic increases took place in the eighties and nineties. Between 1988 and 1994, an average of 11.3% of children ages 6 through 11 and 10.5% of children ages 12 through 19 were obese. This means that over the past few years, the number of obese children is increasing by roughly a half-percentage per year. If you think the word "epidemic" is too dramatic to describe the problem of childhood obesity, consider that this rate of increase is much faster than that of the AIDS "epidemic" which began nearly twenty-five years ago. Today less than 1% of American adults are infected by HIV, the virus that causes AIDS.

WHY OBESITY MATTERS

Does obesity really matter? The huge attention that this problem has received in the media in recent years has created a small but intense backlash. Some claim that the problem of obesity is overblown. This is completely untrue. If anything, obesity, especially among children, is not being taken as seriously as it should be. Moreover, the attention that obesity has received, as we will see, has brought about some significant positive changes in schools, the food industry, and in public policy.

Like smoking, obesity has a profound and broad impact on people's health. A child who begins smoking at age 12 is going to experience the most serious consequences many years later. By contrast, an obese twelve-year-old experiences serious adverse medical, psychological, and social effects of obesity, both as a child and later in adulthood. For many people, obesity is a lifelong problem that manifests itself in different ways throughout the lifespan.

The Economic Impact

These days, no discussion of a significant public health problem is complete without mention of its economic impact. For many people, this may not be the most interesting aspect of the impact of obesity, but it is worth acknowledging up front. Healthcare resources are limited and the cost of caring for patients with obesity and obesity-related diseases is an important measure of the scope of the problem. Unfortunately, there are no reports about healthcare costs specifically for obesity among children. The overall healthcare cost for obesity among both adults and children in the United States is roughly $93 billion annually.[8] This includes the cost of caring for obesity-related diseases such as gallbladder disease and diabetes. This number represents an incredible 9% of all dollars spent on healthcare. The actual amount of money spent on obesity is substantially higher when one considers that Americans spend roughly $33 billion annually on weight-loss products and services.[9] The economic cost of obesity is higher than that of smoking or virtually any other medical problem. Controlling obesity would have a huge impact on overall healthcare costs that are spiraling out of control.

Obesity and the Insulin Resistance Syndrome

It has been known for some time that obesity is much more than a cosmetic issue. It is a significant risk factor for diabetes, high blood pressure, and heart disease. What physicians and researchers are beginning to realize is that the processes through which obesity increases the risk for these serious diseases begin in childhood. In an obese child, many factors, some of which go unrecognized, act together over time to lead to poor adult health. Obesity allows a number of chemical processes in the body to work together and flourish. Over time, these often lead to serious adult diseases. The evidence for this mechanism is increasingly strong and comes in different forms. *Atherosclerosis*, or narrowing of the arteries, is a disease of blood vessels that is responsible for heart disease and other conditions. Children sometimes die unexpectedly, in accidents for example. In such unfortunate circumstances, autopsies of some children as young as five years old have revealed early atherosclerosis. Atherosclerosis of this type is worse in obese children.[10] The seeds of heart disease are therefore planted at a very young age.

The precise way in which obesity in childhood allows serious diseases to develop is the subject of intense research. In 1988 Dr. Gerald Reaven proposed a new theory that provides a "unifying" or single explanation for the causes of hypertension, high cholesterol, diabetes, heart disease, and other conditions.[11] Insulin is a hormone produced by the pancreas that controls blood sugar. When you eat a bag of potato chips, for example, the starch in the potatoes is quickly broken down into simple sugar that enters the bloodstream. Sugar is a form of energy. Some of this energy will be used up quickly. The sugar triggers the release of insulin, whose job is to "mop up" any remaining sugar and help store it in body tissues such as the liver. Excess energy can then be converted to fat. Patients with *type 1 diabetes* (childhood diabetes) produce little or no insulin and do not have the ability to regulate their blood sugar in this way. This is why they require insulin injections.

The ability of insulin to do its job is affected by obesity. For several reasons insulin has more trouble acting to mop up blood sugar and store it in people with a lot of body fat, especially abdominal fat in and around important organs like the liver. This phenomenon is called "insulin resistance." Like a mailman who has more trouble trudging through deep snow than clear streets to do his job, insulin has more trouble trudging through fat to do its job. The phenomenon of resistance to the action of insulin and the diseases associated with it are collectively known as the *insulin resistance syndrome.*

The body responds to insulin resistance by producing more insulin. More of the hormone is produced and circulated in the bloodstream to keep blood sugar levels under control. It is now believed that the higher level of circulating insulin in obese people with insulin resistance causes a great deal of trouble. Insulin is a complex protein that has various effects on different body tissues. It is known to increase salt retention and to increase the strength of nerve impulses to blood vessels, causing them to narrow or "constrict." These are the mechanisms through which insulin resistance is thought to cause high blood pressure. Insulin also influences the development of high cholesterol by promoting production of LDL or "bad" cholesterol and promoting breakdown of HDL or "good" cholesterol.[12]

The mechanism through which obesity and insulin resistance are related to the development of diabetes is relatively easy to understand. Type 2 diabetes (previously known as "adult-onset diabetes"), like type 1 diabetes, is characterized by high, uncontrolled levels of blood sugar. As insulin resistance first develops, blood sugar levels can still be kept under control by the compensatory production of more insulin. As insulin resistance gets progressively worse, eventually the body cannot compensate by producing enough insulin to keep sugar levels under control. In other words, there comes a point where insulin resistance cannot be overcome. At this point, blood sugar levels begin to rise and patients are diagnosed with type 2 diabetes. Type 2 diabetes, like type 1 diabetes, has serious complications.

Unlike diabetes, high blood pressure and high cholesterol do not usually cause any symptoms. High blood pressure, for example, has been often called a "silent killer." Diabetes, high blood pressure, and high cholesterol are known as *cardiovascular risk factors*. They promote the development of atherosclerosis in different blood vessels in the body. Atherosclerosis can develop in the arteries supplying the heart muscle itself that are known as the *coronary arteries*. If severe enough, the narrowing of the coronary arteries can cut off blood supply to the heart. The heart muscle begins to die. This is what takes place during a "heart attack." In a similar way, atherosclerosis can cause strokes and disease of the blood vessels of the limbs known as *peripheral vascular disease*.

Other important cardiovascular risk factors include smoking and a strong family history of heart disease. The more risk factors one has, the greater the likelihood of development of atherosclerosis and the greater the cardiovascular risk in the long term. This leads us to the end of an important chain of events that begins with obesity. Obesity promotes insulin resistance. Insulin resistance allows many important cardiovascular risk factors to develop. These risk factors promote atherosclerosis. As atherosclerosis progresses in severity, it can cause severe, even fatal cardiovascular disease. This is why researchers are focused on better understanding the precise links in this chain and how to slow down or disrupt the process.

Medical Complications of Obesity

An obese child, especially one with a family history of obesity, is likely to become an obese adult. In fact, 80% of children ages 10 to 14 with at least one obese parent become obese adults.[13] Obesity has a significant impact on both the physical and the psychological well-being of children that continues into adulthood.

The term "adult-onset diabetes" has been replaced by "type 2 diabetes" because so many children are developing what used to be an almost exclusively adult problem. As it progresses, insulin resistance eventually makes it difficult or impossible for the body to control blood sugar levels. High blood sugar that cannot normally be controlled without medication is the hallmark of diabetes. Insulin resistance frequently develops among obese, inactive adults. The time between the onset of insulin resistance and the point at which it cannot be overcome to keep blood sugar in check can take several years or even decades. As obesity has become much more common among young children, so has insulin resistance. The process through which diabetes develops, therefore, is occurring earlier and earlier.

The number of children diagnosed with type 2 diabetes increased tenfold between 1982 and 1992 and continues to soar.[14] Not long ago, nearly all cases of diabetes among children were type 1. Now nearly half are type 2.[15] The implications are highly serious. Type 2 diabetes worsens over time. Blood sugar becomes more and more difficult to control and requires an increasing number of and increasing doses of medications. High blood sugar makes people fatigued, thirsty, and hungry. Blurry vision is common. More important than just feeling unwell are the long-term complications of diabetes including kidney failure, blindness, and heart disease. An adult diagnosed with type 2 diabetes at age 50 may suffer these consequences in his or her sixties or seventies. A fifteen-year-old diagnosed with type 2 diabetes may require kidney dialysis or suffer a heart attack in his thirties or forties—the prime of his life.

Today, diseases other than type 2 diabetes that are associated with insulin resistance, including high blood pressure and high cholesterol, are being more frequently diagnosed among children. Obesity is placing a large number of children at increased cardiovascular risk. This is why the grim prospect of children not outliving their parents is being sounded as an alarm. A Harvard study that followed individuals beginning at ages 13 to 18 over the course of fifty years revealed that obese boys were twice as likely to die from heart disease as normal-weight boys.[16] In fact, obesity that develops in adolescence places an individual at greater risk of early death than obesity that develops in adulthood.

Many people know the association of obesity with cardiovascular risk. The stereotypical "heart attack waiting to happen" is thought to refer to an obese, middle-aged man who eats poorly and doesn't exercise. Most people are not aware, however, of the link between obesity and other medical illnesses.

Obesity is not the only serious chronic disease that is becoming increasingly common among children. Asthma is a chronic inflammation of the airways in and outside the lungs that causes symptoms of shortness of breath, chronic cough, wheezing, and chest tightness. Like the number of obese children, the number of children with asthma, especially severe asthma, has been increasing steadily over the past ten years. Physicians started to speculate about a link between the two diseases some time ago. In my own practice, in the mid-1990s I started to notice anecdotally that among children with asthma, overweight and obese children seemed to suffer more. They required a larger number of and higher doses of asthma medications. Their symptoms were more severe and they required hospitalization for asthma more often. Today, obesity is a well-established risk factor for asthma.[17] Not only are obese children and adults more likely to develop asthma than normal-weight individuals, but their asthma is likely to be severe. The encouraging news is that weight loss in obese, asthmatic patients significantly reduces the severity of asthma.[18] How obesity influences asthma risk and severity is not entirely clear. Several explanations have been proposed. One possibility is that excess body fat makes it more difficult to move large volumes of air in and out of the lungs, worsening shortness of breath. Obese children and adults are also more likely to suffer from acid reflux (heartburn). Acid reflux, in turn, is known to make asthma more severe. Other possible explanations involve the immune system and sex hormones.[19]

About 15% of children snore. Sometimes snoring is inconsequential. Often, snoring is a symptom of *sleep-disordered breathing*, a phenomenon characterized by decreased flow of air in and out of the lungs while sleeping, or even episodes of complete stoppage of breathing for several seconds, known as *apnea*. About 1% to 3% of all children have sleep-disordered breathing. Obesity is a significant risk factor: 26% to 33% of obese children have sleep-disordered breathing.[20] Snoring may be no more than a nuisance to a child or his family, but the other symptoms of sleep-disordered breathing are severe. Affected children sleep poorly. They have trouble getting to bed and awaken frequently at night. As a result they usually feel tired or sleepy in the daytime. Many need naps. This has an obvious impact on how well they do in school. It's hard for a child to pay attention to his teacher, for example, when he keeps falling asleep.

Obesity is related to other, less common medical complications both among children and adults. Obese children are at greater risk of bone problems including *Blount's disease*, a disease characterized by bending or bowing of the legs. Apart from insulin resistance and its associated conditions and diseases affecting breathing, the most devastating complications of obesity are psychological and social. Like the complications of insulin resistance syndrome, the psychological and social complications of obesity begin in childhood and manifest in different ways throughout life.

The Psychological and Social Consequences for Children

The most surprising aspect of all the attention that is being paid to the problem of obesity in the news media is the lack of emphasis on how obesity affects psychological and social well-being. Most media coverage about obesity focuses on its rising prevalence among children and the ways to fight it. When consequences are discussed, the emphasis is upon diabetes and heart disease. It's almost as if the "psychosocial" impact of obesity is a taboo subject. By contrast, behavioral scientists and physicians have written a great deal about this aspect of the disease. The impact of obesity upon a child's mental health and immediate and future social life is every bit as important as the impact on physical health.

The psychosocial impact of obesity upon children is mainly the result of how such children are perceived by their peers and adults. Overweight and obese children are subjected to both subtle and blatant forms of isolation, unfairness, and cruelty. The impact is profound and can last a lifetime. Despite the increasing number of obese children, our society continues to place a supreme value on thinness. There is a vast number of books on the market about overcoming obesity or overcoming eating disorders such as anorexia nervosa. Sincere stories of what it's like to be an overweight or obese child, however, are surprisingly rare.

Judy Blume is a prominent author of children's books. One of the best accounts of the life of an overweight child can be found in her 1974 book, *Blubber*. It tells the story of Linda, an overweight fifth-grader, who is asked to give a class presentation about a mammal of her choice. She chooses the whale and includes a description of whale blubber and its various commercial uses. From that point on, she receives the nickname "Blubber" and becomes the target of teasing and cruel pranks. One of her classmates invents this rhyme:[21]

> Oh, what a riot
> Blubber's on a diet
> I wonder what's the matter
> I think she's getting fatter
> And fatter
> And fatter
> And fatter
> Pop!

It gets worse. At one point Linda's Halloween costume is pulled off by other girls who proceed to strip her down to her underwear. At another point, Linda is held down by her classmates and force-fed a chocolate-covered ant. Interestingly, Linda weighs 91 lbs. and in 1974 this was considered to be far too much. Blume never reveals Linda's height in the book, but there is nothing to indicate that she is either shorter or taller than average. Today, 91 lbs. is only just above the 50th percentile of weight for eleven-year-old girls (fifth-graders). Basically, by today's standards, "Blubber" would most likely be pretty average.

Some of Judy Blume's books have been banned from school libraries and classrooms because they deal with supposedly "controversial" themes like puberty or because they include adult language. *Blubber* has also been subjected to censorship. What's controversial about it? Blume believes that adults are bothered by how cruel children can be to each other.[22] Banning the book is a good way to sweep the problem under the rug.

Blubber is pure fiction. In real life, obese children sometimes suffer worse at the hands of other children and adults. In 1999 Gina Score, an obese fourteen-year-old girl, was sent to a juvenile detention camp for petty theft. Physical workouts were a big part of camp activities. On a hot day, Gina, who weighed 224 lbs., was forced to participate in a 2.7-mile run. She quickly fell behind the other teens, but the camp instructors forced her to continue. After a while she collapsed and turned pale. She began frothing from the mouth. The adult instructors sat by drinking soda, ridiculing Gina, and accusing her of faking. She lay there for four hours before an ambulance was called. Several of her internal organs failed. She died shortly thereafter.[23]

A negative perception of overweight and obese children by other children and adults is a well-documented and widespread phenomenon. Many years ago, T. A. Wadden and A. J. Stunkard studied the perception of obese children among children ages 6 and younger.[24] Children were shown drawings of obese children as well as silhouettes of children with various handicaps such as missing limbs or facial disfigurement. The obese children were rated as the least likable. Obese children were described as lazy, dirty, stupid, and ugly as well as cheats and liars. This perception was uniform among different racial and ethnic groups. Kids therefore not only ridicule the physical attributes of obese children but for some reason also seem to judge their characters harshly.

What inspires such intense contempt especially at such a young age? No one really knows. Though in some cultures and in some groups obesity is viewed more favorably than in others, obese people in general have been treated contemptuously for a very long time. Pope Gregory included gluttony among the seven deadly sins in the sixth century, probably because both gluttony and obesity were viewed as connected and hence worthy of disgust. There might be more to it than that. There may be something visceral or ingrained within all of us that provokes a negative reaction toward the obese. This would explain why even very young children exercise prejudice.

Another contributing explanation for why obese children are mistreated by other children may be that discrimination on the basis of weight is still acceptable in our society. The vast majority of Americans believe it is unfair to mistreat people on the basis of race, religion, ethnicity, or sex. Children are also taught repeatedly by parents, teachers, and the media that these forms of discrimination are wrong. Such tolerance does not seem to extend to obese children. There are public service announcements on television promoting acceptance of people of different races but none to discourage discrimination against the obese. No wonder obesity has been called "the last bastion of prejudice."[25]

The psychological impact of prejudice of the type I've described is devastating. Obese children and adolescents have a much more negative body image than children of normal weight and are more likely to suffer from low self-esteem.[26] This extends into adulthood. In fact, the more often a child is teased about weight and shape while growing up, the more dissatisfied she will be as an adult.[27] A negative body image and low self-esteem are more common among obese girls than among obese boys.[28] Severely obese girls have lower self-esteem than moderately obese girls.[29] Obese African American girls, however, are less likely to have low self-esteem than their white or Latina counterparts.

Some obese children have normal self-esteem and have been studied to determine how their attitudes differ from those of other obese children. They appear to have two coping mechanisms.[30] First, they diminish the importance of activities in which they do not or cannot excel and place more emphasis on other things. An obese twelve-year-old boy, for example, may describe his lack of ability or lack of interest in sports as completely unimportant in relation to his skill with computers. Some obese children also cope by having a somewhat distorted body image. The same obese boy may describe himself as just a bit stocky or "well built" rather than obese, or under-estimate his size in relation to his peers.

A few studies have shown that obese children are more likely to suffer from serious psychiatric disorders than other children. A 1999 study revealed higher rates of mood disorders and anxiety among overweight girls than normal-weight girls.[31] Depression is more common among children seeking treatment for obesity than among other children.[32] Behavior problems such as acting out in school are also more common among obese ten- to sixteen-year-olds than among other children.[33] Other studies have disputed the association of obesity with psychiatric disorders. It is also not clear whether obese children are somehow predisposed to psychiatric problems, or if being targeted by other children and even adults results in such problems.

The Psychological and Social Impact in Adulthood

Many obese children grow up to be normal-weight adults; many do not. Even many normal-weight adults who were obese as children continue to bear the burden of obesity in the form of low self-esteem or distorted body image. The situation is far worse among people for whom obesity is a lifelong problem. In addition to caring for children in my role as the clinical director of the Weight Management and Wellness Center at the Children's Hospital of Pittsburgh, I do treat many obese adults in my family practice. Obesity-related diseases such as diabetes and hypertension are the focus of treatment. Rarely does a discussion of the psychosocial impact of obesity come up. In fact, none of my obese adult patients has ever complained about being discriminated against for being obese. This may be because discrimi-nation against obese adults is subtler than discrimination against obese children. I've observed it firsthand.

In my neighborhood a busy city bus carries commuters to work and students to school. The bus fills up quickly. An obese woman boards the bus every morning. She is large but not large enough to require two seats. As the bus gets more crowded, people find a seat anywhere except next to the obese woman. When the seats run out, people decide to stand rather than sit next to her. Nobody sits next to the obese woman the whole trip. Though she probably had the most comfortable ride on the bus, I believe the fact that no one sits next to her is a subtle, perhaps even unconscious expression of how people react to obesity. Prejudice against the obese in adulthood may be subtle, but its impact is huge.

Discrimination against the obese in educational settings has been documented in college admissions. Nearly forty years ago, it was found that obese high school students were less likely to be accepted to college than their normal-weight peers despite equivalent qualifications.[34] Obese young women were more likely to suffer this type of discrimination than obese young men. Discrimination in educational settings persists. One of the reasons obese women are less likely to be accepted is that they receive less financial support from their parents than normal-weight daughters.[35] It appears that discrimination begins at home.

Discrimination against obese adults has been well documented in the workplace, in educational settings, and even within the healthcare system. Studies that use simulated descriptions of employees and managers of different weights showed a significant bias. One survey revealed that, based on fictitious descriptions of female employees who differed by weight, young women expressed the greatest desire to work with thin women and the least desire to work with obese women.[36] Another study used simulations of prospective employees interviewing for jobs. The study, while controlling for other factors, revealed that obese candidates were less likely than normal-weight candidates to be recommended for public sales jobs and more likely to be recommended for jobs with little or no face-to-face contact. The degree of this bias was stronger against obese female than obese male candidates.[37] Obese employees are widely perceived as lazy, lacking self-discipline, less conscientious, less competent, sloppy, and emotionally unstable.[38]

These workplace biases have a significant impact upon prospects for advancement and income. Obese women, for example, earn 12% less than normal-weight women.[39] Overall, obese men do not earn less than normal-weight men, but earn less in some managerial and professional occupations.[40]

Discrimination against the obese takes place in a number of other different settings and in a variety of forms. Obese women, for example, are less likely to marry than normal-weight women.[41]

As a physician, what I find most disturbing is the prejudice that the obese face from members of my own profession. A survey of four hundred family physicians in 1982 revealed shocking attitudes toward obese patients.[42] Physicians were asked to identify problems or types of patients that provoked negative feelings and attitudes. Obese patients, along with alcoholics, drug addicts, and the mentally ill, were among the groups identified. In the same survey, obesity was associated with poor hygiene, hostility, and dishonesty. Physicians make character judgments about obese patients, therefore, that are similar to the judgments that children make about their obese peers. Similar attitudes have been reported among medical students and nurses: 24% of nurses find caring for an obese patient repulsive, and 12% prefer not to touch obese patients.[43] Medical students describe obese patients as worthless, unpleasant, ugly, and lacking self-control.[44] These attitudes were found in older studies, but there is little evidence to suggest that things have improved. Moreover, negative attitudes manifest themselves in extremely important ways. For example, 17% of physicians are reluctant to provide pelvic examinations to obese women.[45] Obese women themselves are less likely to seek gynecologic care. The net result is that the quality of care that obese women receive is inferior partly as a result of the negative attitudes of the people who ought to care most.

THE CAUSES OF CHILDHOOD OBESITY

Now that you have more understanding of the repercussions of the problem, it is time to turn to the causes of childhood obesity. Like the consequences of obesity, the causes are intricate and varied. Childhood obesity is the end result of a complex interaction among genetic and environmental factors. In short, no single factor makes a child obese. A very small number of children have inherited or acquired conditions that are responsible for their obesity. It is also true that some healthy children are genetically predisposed to become obese. Genetics, however, cannot explain the obesity epidemic in America today. While obesity rates among children are skyrocketing, the gene pool has been relatively stable. This means the environment in which children live is the place to look for causes of the obesity epidemic. Even a child predisposed to becoming obese can remain thinner in the right environment.

Within the environment there are as many different suspects as causes of childhood obesity. After much research, I've come up with a short list of the five most important: sweetened (regular) soft drinks; fast food; television; physical inactivity; and changing or harmful family meal patterns and feeding practices. The rest of the first half of this book is devoted to understanding and targeting these culprits.

Chapter Two

"Liquid Candy":
Kids Raised on Soft Drinks

I made an interesting discovery on a hot day last summer while driving between Pittsburgh and Washington, DC. I needed a boost of caffeine and decided to stop along the way at one of those huge rest stops on the Interstate highway. Outside was a row of ten self-serve gas pumps with speakers broadcasting messages beckoning customers to come inside for a hot dog and fries. Inside, hungry travelers had a choice of a couple of fast-food outlets and a snack and gift shop. I just wanted a diet soda with caffeine—something to keep me awake for the rest of the trip. Hot coffee on a hot day didn't strike me as very appealing. The shop was well stocked with maps, cigarettes, candy, and travel necessities such as sunscreen. The drinks were housed in three huge refrigerated display cases in the back. The variety was amazing. The big names in soft drinks were, as expected, well represented. I also found large colorful bottles of iced tea, a complete range of blue and green sports drinks (that would probably glow in the dark with the lights shut off), and cartons of milk in a variety of flavors. One entire display case was devoted to juice in one form or another—bottles of orange juice, vegetable drinks, and drinks that resembled real juice in some ways but weren't real. A small section contained three or four types of bottled water, including flavored varieties. There was also a section of "energy" drinks. These came in menacing, aggressive-looking shiny metal cans and cost more than two dollars each.

I found soda only in 20 oz. bottles. I really didn't want that much, so I looked around for a 12 oz. can. No luck. Taking in the full breadth of the more than one hundred different drinks on display, I realized that besides a few small cans of energy drinks, there were no cans of anything at all. Did companies suddenly abandon the 12 oz. can? I grabbed a cold 20 oz. bottle of water. "Do you not sell any 12 oz. cans of pop?" I asked the cashier.

"We used to sell them. I don't know. I guess they're not making so many of them anymore. I guess people just want the big bottles now," she replied. Her assessment was correct. I am part of the older segment of Generation X and have watched soft drink containers grow up into the tall missiles sold everywhere today. I grew up in Canada where in the late 1970s and early 1980s kids complained that our soft drink cans were only 284 ml or 10 oz. while across the border the standard size was 12 oz. The complaining must have worked. By the time I was in high school, 12 oz. became standard in Canada and the path to gargantuan sizes had been well established.

Are we all just getting thirstier? How much soda are today's children drinking? Why are they drinking so much and why does it matter?

THE RISE OF THE CARBONATED BEVERAGE

The rise of the carbonated beverage is a complex phenomenon with many driving forces. Soft drinks are, of course, everywhere. You can buy them in grocery stores, from vending machines, institutional cafeterias, gas stations, convenience stores, movie theaters, fast-food restaurants, department stores, national parks, campgrounds, museums, and sporting venues. Widespread availability has without a doubt led to greater consumption.

Availability and consumption, however, have not always spurred sales for other types of foods. Take the case of chocolate. It's also everywhere and seemingly in everything. There's chocolate milk and milkshakes, candy bars, cakes, cookies, and ice cream, to name a few options. Just about everything edible has at one point been creatively or foolishly covered in chocolate. Chocolate candy, packaged chocolate cakes and cookies, and chocolate drinks are often sold in the same places as soft drinks. Unexpectedly, per capita consumption of cocoa (from which chocolate is made) in the United States actually declined in the early 1990s before recovering slightly in the late 1990s. The average American consumed roughly the same amount of chocolate in 2000 (4.6–4.7lbs./year) as he or she did in 1990.[1] Unlike the case of soft drinks, selling chocolate everywhere has not increased Americans' taste for it. Europeans eat far more of it and sometimes in strange ways. A restaurant in the Ukraine, for example, is doing a booming business selling chocolate-covered pork fat![2]

The rise in both availability and consumption of soft drinks is related to the evolving role they have played in our lives. This role has always been defined by the companies that make soft drinks. A history lesson is useful in this regard. Soft drinks have been around for hundreds of years in one form or another. As early as 1676 the Compagnie de Limonadiers (Lemonade Vendors' Company) began selling cups of lemon juice, water, and honey in Paris as a safe form of rejuvenation.[3] In the eighteenth century, the English chemist Joseph Priestley produced the first glass of drinkable carbonated water. Carbonated water and sugar, the basic recipe for all soft drinks, was born two hundred years ago. John Matthews patented a machine for making carbonated water in 1832. Soda fountains became popular in America quickly thereafter. Interestingly, soda concoctions were first promoted for their health benefits and frequently included exotic ingredients such as dandelions and birch bark. Drug stores were the principal vendors of soda. In fact, Coca-Cola was invented by a pharmacist.[4]

With the mass production of glass bottles and the invention of tight seals in the late 1800s and early 1900s, soft drinks became portable and widely available. Children were important consumers of soft drinks even then. On its "Heritage" Web site, the Coca-Cola Company includes a collection of stories from customers who have enjoyed its product dating back a hundred years. Most of the stories are about parents buying their then young children Coke as a special but affordable treat.[5]

Gradually soft drinks evolved from health-promoting tonics to special treats and finally to a big part of people's diets. Soaring consumption is described in a report by Dr. Michael Jacobson, "Liquid Candy: How Soft Drinks Are Harming Americans' Health."[6] Per capita soft drink consumption in the United States increased almost sixfold between 1947 and 1997 to reach 576 12 oz. servings per person per year. Retail sales of soft drinks totaled nearly $64 billion in 2003.[7] Surveys have shown that up to 85% of schoolchildren consume at least one 12 oz. soft drink daily; 20% consume four or more servings the same size.[8] The heaviest drinkers are boys aged 12 to 19 who consume a remarkable average of 28.5 oz. daily (compared with 20.4 oz. daily for girls the same age).[9]

As Americans' thirst for soft drinks has increased, soft drinks have displaced other drinks from the diet. Per capita total consumption of milk, for example, actually fell from 269.1 pounds per person in 1970 to 209.7 pounds in 1995 and continues to fall rapidly. The percentage of children, especially teenagers, drinking at least some milk is declining sharply. In 1977–78, 22% of girls aged 14–17, for example, consumed at least some milk on any given day. This dropped to just 9% between 1994 and 1998.[10]

WHAT SOFT DRINKS DO TO CHILDREN

Children are drinking soft drinks like never before. So what? If each American child had a soft drink once in a while it would certainly not be a problem. Today's soda-drinking kids, however, suffer in a big way. Soft drinks do many bad things to children, and medical research is still uncovering more. Just as doctors and public health officials have for years carefully produced charts and documents to summarize the incredible number of serious effects of cigarette smoking, it is worthwhile to describe in detail what is known about the adverse health effects of drinking so much "liquid candy."

Obesity

Obesity is the most important and most obvious impact of drinking huge quantities of soft drinks. The evidence is conclusive. In a Massachusetts study, 548 children (with an average age of eleven) were followed for nineteen months to determine the impact of soft drinks on body weight.[11] Each serving of soft drink a child drank per day was associated with an increase in body mass index of 0.24 kg/m^2. The researchers made sure that other factors like growth, other parts of the diet, and lifestyle (e.g., television watching) could not explain the results. To put it more simply, consider two boys, each aged 11 with a height of 4'10" and a weight of 100 lbs., and maturing at the same rate. One drinks one 12 oz. can of regular soda per day; the other, two cans a day. At the end of nineteen months, if the first boy were 5'5" and 133 lbs., the second would be 5'5" and roughly 2 lbs. heavier. At first, two pounds doesn't sound like a big problem. Imagine, however, that the second boy continues to gain weight at a rate that is two pounds higher than the first every nineteen months. It isn't hard to imagine that the second boy will weigh significantly more when he becomes an adult. Not surprisingly, the Massachusetts researchers found that each additional serving of soft drink increases a child's odds of becoming obese by an incredible 60%.

You might think that the ability to make kids fat isn't unique to soft drinks. After all, peanuts will make a child overweight or obese if he or she eats enough of them. Soft drinks, however, have some interesting properties that make them especially potent. They are laden with sugar—usually in the form of high-fructose corn syrup. A 12 oz. can of regular soft drink contains the equivalent of ten teaspoons of sugar. Can you imagine adding ten teaspoons of sugar to a cup of coffee or tea? This brings us to another important property. Soft drinks, like other junk foods, have been criticized for providing "empty calories," which means that they provide calories without any other nutrients. I also call these "silent" calories. People just don't realize how many calories they are taking in and, afterward, don't really "feel" the extra calories.

Normally, most foods we eat in excess stimulate what is known as an involuntary "compensatory response." An office worker who eats a big piece of cake at 10:30 AM is probably going to eat less at lunch than usual, even if she doesn't specifically plan it. Dr. Richard Mattes has shown that soft drinks (among other drinks) don't stimulate a compensatory response.[12] In other words, if that same office worker had a 20 oz. bottle of soda at 10:30 AM, eating his or her usual lunch would feel completely normal. Children have even less ability to "compensate" for calories from soft drinks than adults. Not only do they have the same lack of *involuntary* compensatory response as adults, but they also have less knowledge of nutrition and don't think about how many calories they are taking in. After drinking soft drinks, children don't *voluntarily* compensate by eating less food at other times either.

Nutritional labels on soft drink containers that indicate the proper serving size do not seem to influence children. First of all, even adults are frequently confused by serving sizes recommended on labels.[13] Imagine how confusing they are for kids. The labels on soft drinks are also frequently inconsistent. A 12 oz. can of soft drink bears a label describing its contents as one serving. You can find lots of tall 24 oz. bottles of soft drinks now in convenience stores. These are popular with children[14] and their labels describe the contents as three, not two, servings (i.e., 8 oz. rather than 12 oz. per serving). Even a rare, health-conscious child who pays attention to food labels would likely be left wondering about the proper serving size. Furthermore, there is evidence that food portion size in general influences how much children eat.[15] The bigger the portions they receive, the more they take in. Give a child a 16 oz. bottle of soft drink and he may drink 12 oz. at one time. Give him a 20 oz. bottle and he may drink 15 oz. at one time.

Diabetes

Diabetes is a serious disease affecting more than eighteen million Americans. Complications include heart disease, blindness, and amputations. Most affected patients have type 2 diabetes, or what used to be called "adult-onset" diabetes. Sadly, diabetes and obesity are closely linked. As discussed in chapter 1, the huge rise in the number of very obese children has meant that type 2 diabetes no longer affects only adults. It is now being diagnosed in children as young as ten. It isn't surprising that soft drinks, which are linked to obesity, are also linked to diabetes. A recent study showed that women who drank at least one soft drink a day were 85% more likely to develop type 2 diabetes than women who drank less.[16] Though only adults were studied, it is reasonable to assume that soft drinks also increase the risk of diabetes in children.

Dental Caries

Many of the children in my practice have terrible teeth. I will often find a six-year-old with a mouth full of erosions, cavities, infection, and gum disease. There is an epidemic of rotten teeth among America's children, especially poor and minority childen.[17] The causes include inadequate brushing, lack of access to dental care especially among the poor, and, of course, sugar. Sugar is everywhere in a child's world. Soft drinks are the leading source. They also contain lots of acid. Sugar and acid in combination have been shown to accelerate tooth decay. The more soft drinks a child consumes, the more cavities they are likely to develop.[18] Even more disturbing, fluoride, which is found in many municipal water supplies and in toothpaste, does not protect teeth from the erosive effect of soft drinks.[19] In other words, soft drinks can destroy teeth like no other food.

Bones

There are a number of reports in the medical literature linking soft drink consumption to low bone density (i.e., weak bones) and fractures in both children and adults. This is still controversial. Active high school girls who drink soft drinks regularly are three times more likely to report having had a bone fracture than girls who don't drink soft drinks.[20] A more recent study found that the higher the soft drink consumption among girls aged 12 to 15, the lower the density of their heel bones.[21] No such relationship was found in boys. At this time there just isn't enough information to draw firm conclusions about soft drinks and bone health. There is probably nothing special about soft drinks that weaken bones. Children who drink plenty of soft drinks drink less milk. Milk is rich in calcium, which is necessary for building strong bones during childhood and adolescence. Low bone density later in life (osteoporosis) is certainly associated with fractures and disability. Children who take in little calcium, therefore, may pay a huge price later.

Effect of Caffeine

Caffeine is a well-known stimulant drug and is found in the majority of soft drinks. It is linked to restlessness, headaches, nausea, and insomnia in children.[22] A 2004 study found a relationship between consumption of caffeinated soft drinks and high blood pressure in African American teens.[23] Many questions about the overall effect of caffeine in soft drinks upon children, however, have yet to be explored.

What about Diet and Caffeine-Free Soft Drinks?

Some people are concerned about the potential adverse effects of artificial sweeteners. No *conclusive* evidence of harm from artificial sweeteners currently used in diet drinks exists. What is certain is that calorie-free and calorie-reduced soft drinks are widely available and are not associated with obesity. Caffeine-free soft drinks, though not as widely available as diet drinks, do not have the stimulant side effects of caffeinated drinks. The problem is that children generally do not like or purchase these alternatives.[24] Diet drinks are heavily promoted to health-conscious adults. Kids just don't seem to have a taste for them. Throughout this book, when I refer to "soft drinks," I mean the regular, sweetened variety.

HOW KIDS GOT HOOKED

It would be terrific if kids would just drink less or give up soft drinks completely. Let me tell you as parents what you're up against. Soft drinks have become a major part of children's diets through successful marketing. Foods and drinks have been marketed to children for generations. Television is an important medium. It is estimated that children view an average of forty thousand television commercials a year.[25] More than half are for foods and drinks that are high in fat or sugar or both. Young children are especially vulnerable to the influence of commercials. Unlike older children and adults who "tune out" to some degree during commercials, young children, including preschoolers, remain as attentive as during scheduled programming.[26] Drs. Dina Borzekowski and Thomas Robinson describe the effect of television commercials on children's food preferences in an elegant study.[27] Forty-six two- to six-year-old children were randomly assigned to watch a cartoon, either with or without embedded television commercials. When questioned immediately afterward, children exposed to the commercials preferred the brands of juice, sandwich bread, doughnuts, and candy they had just seen over other brands. Even brief exposure to commercials, therefore, has an impact on children. One can only imagine the impact of forty thousand commercials a year, many of which are repeated over and over again to reinforce their message.

Of course, not all the commercials children watch are for soft drinks. In fact, the Coca-Cola Company has recently adopted a policy of not directly marketing to children under twelve. This is a step in the right direction. But children under twelve certainly have plenty of opportunities to be tempted by soft drinks. Even on television, children themselves are frequently featured in soft drink commercials, often skateboarding or being active in some other way. The clever use of pop icons is hard to miss. Professional basketball players and pop stars rejuvenate themselves with soda after working up a sweat. Soft drink commercials, like commercials for other products, are undoubtedly designed to have a huge impact on young children.

Television is only one and probably not the most effective way in which soft drink companies reach children. A great deal of attention has been focused recently upon banning soft drinks in schools to curb the obesity epidemic. This is a growing movement and is generally a good idea. As recently as the year 2000, however, soft drink vending machines were found in 94.9% of high schools, 62% of middle schools, and 26.3% of elementary schools.[28]

How did soft drinks develop such a strong presence in schools? The US Department of Agriculture has strict nutritional guidelines for what types of foods can be sold in school cafeterias as part of school lunch programs. These standards, however, do not apply to foods sold in school snack bars and vending machines. Most of these "competitive foods" (i.e., foods that compete with USDA-regulated school lunches), including soft drinks, are of low nutritional value.[29] Several state and local school authorities have regulations prohibiting the sale of soft drinks between the start of the school day and the end of the last meal period or in specific locations such as the cafeteria. The rules are frequently broken. A survey in Minnesota, where such rules are supposed to be in place, revealed that among fifty-five high schools, 95% left vending machines unlocked sometime during the day and that 29% left them unlocked all day. Sixty percent of vending machines were located in the school cafeteria.[30] Moreover, companies have also bypassed the rules prohibiting *sales* during lunch periods in some schools by giving children soft drinks *free* with lunch.[31]

The keys to understanding the widespread availability of soft drinks in schools and the lax enforcement of rules restricting sales are the contracts, known as "pouring rights," that schools and school districts sign with soft drink companies. One soft drink company becomes the exclusive vendor for a school or district. Public schools and school districts are facing financial hardship across the country owing in part to cuts in local funding and unreliable funding from state and federal sources.[32] Exclusive pouring rights contracts have become an important source of revenue for schools. The Associated Press contends that Coca-Cola itself has pouring rights contracts with more than six thousand of the fourteen thousand school districts in the United States.[33] A large school district in Colorado, for example, signed a ten-year $8 million deal with Coca-Cola in the late 1990s.[34] One school district in Texas negotiated a $19 million contract.[35] Some deals are even bigger.

Pouring rights contracts have four principal characteristics.[36] First, schools are rewarded financially when children drink more. This provides a disincentive to restricting the sale of soft drinks. According to a 1999 *Harper's* magazine article, some schools and school districts have actually been "pushing" soft drinks on children for this reason.[37] Some school officials have simply failed to realize that the long-term impact upon the health of students is certainly not worth the brief infusion of cash that comes with pouring rights contracts.

The second important feature of pouring rights contracts includes advertising and promotion of soda products in school and at school-related activities. Soft drink advertising takes the form of free distribution of promotional items like hats, T-shirts, and scoreboards bearing soft drink logos. Pepsi advertises on Channel One, a television network that broadcasts to twelve thousand schools, reaching millions of children.[38] Soft drink companies frequently distribute prizes to students at promotional events—everything from samples of their products to automobiles. The goal is to build brand loyalty so that children will shun competitors' products. This can be taken to extremes. In 1998 Greenbriar High School in Georgia held a "Coke in Education Day."[39] Greenbriar was participating in a contest to win a $10,000 prize awarded to the school with the best idea for marketing Coke discount cards. The day's events included the baking of a Coke cake by home economics students. In another key event, all twelve hundred of the school's students were asked to line up in the parking lot to spell out the word "Coke" as Coke executives looked on. While photographers captured the spectacle, a high school senior unashamedly unveiled his Pepsi T-shirt. The school principal suspended him promptly for misbehaving, and more important, for potentially costing the school a lot of money.

The third feature of pouring rights contracts is the right of soft drink companies to determine where and how products are sold. A 1998 contract between a school district in Syracuse, New York, and Coca-Cola, for example, stipulates that the company must be allowed to place a minimum of 135 vending machines in schools.[40] In most contracts, vending machine locations must be agreed to by the soft drink company.

Finally, pouring rights contracts are negotiated in an unexpected way. Nutritionists and other health professionals are normally not involved. The majority of schools view the contracts as simply business transactions from which they can benefit financially. In fact, some schools have hired consultants to help them negotiate the best deals. Nutrition and health are never on the agenda of topics to be discussed.

The way soft drinks are marketed to kids old enough to drink from a cup, can, glass, or plastic bottle is disturbing enough. Soft drink companies have also extended their reach to an even more vulnerable group. One of my patients recently brought her two children, a five-year-old daughter and a twelve-month-old son, in for a checkup. I started to examine the five-year-old when the baby started to cry. His mother reached into her purse, pulled out a baby bottle, and stuck it promptly in his mouth. The bottle was full of cola. Cola is, of course, about as inappropriate a baby food as one can imagine. Feeding infants soft drinks in baby bottles, however, is more common than I first realized. According to *USA Today*, Pepsi, Dr. Pepper, and Seven-Up have licensed their logos to Munchkin Bottling Inc., one of America's largest baby bottle manufacturers.[41] The logos work. Babies fed with logo-bearing bottles are four times more likely to receive soft drinks than babies fed with ordinary bottles.[42]

Chapter Three

Fast-Food Epidemic

S oft drinks and fast food go hand in hand. Both are everywhere. Stop at a fast-food restaurant and the question "What would you like to drink with that?" rolls spontaneously off the food server's tongue. Fast food means different things to different people. A standard definition is helpful. Fast food is food purchased or eaten outside the home that is inexpensive (usually well under $10 per person per meal); that is prepared, served, and eaten quickly; and that is available in an identical or nearly identical form from franchised outlets. This definition excludes food from what have come to be known as *fast casual* restaurants. These more upscale places, such as Boston Market and Panera Bread Co., generally offer healthier meals at higher prices. Most fast food sold in traditional outlets (e.g., McDonald's and Burger King) is high in fat and calories. Not everything these places sell, however, is unhealthy. Subway, for example, offers a number of healthy sandwich choices. Even the big burger chains now offer healthier alternatives such as salads. From here on, when I refer to fast food, I mean the items that form the "core" of the business: burgers, french fries, soft drinks and shakes, chicken nuggets, fried chicken, ice cream, and packaged cakes. Children love these foods.

Fast food has certainly received a lot of negative press lately. Eric Schlosser's superb book *Fast Food Nation*[1] outlines in detail the origins of the fast-food business as well as the exploitation of workers in the food-processing industry and other information regarding fast-food restaurant employees and franchise owners. Schlosser also discloses the way fast food is "designed" and marketed. More recently, the film *Supersize Me* reveals the impact of a fast-food diet on a healthy young adult. My purpose here is to tell you about what fast food does to children and why it is so hard for them to resist. I'm not going to start, however, by telling you about the evils of fast food, the "Dark Side of the All-American Meal," as Schlosser so eloquently subtitled his book. I recently got a glimpse of the love affair between children and fast food. Here is a story about how beautiful fast food can be.

Arriving at Pittsburgh International Airport is like landing in a shopping mall. It's an extravagant facility full of shops and restaurants in every direction. The "Airmall" boasts that everything is available at "regular mall prices." Indeed, before airport security was tightened after 9/11, the Airmall was a popular shopping destination even among Pittsburghers with no flight to catch. Among the chain stores like the Gap and Sharper Image are all kinds of fast- and fast-casual food restaurants. Food dominates the airport's massive retail space. You'll find coffee, bagels, pizza, Chinese food, submarine sandwiches, beer, croissants, candy, and not one but two McDonald's.

I never had a huge taste for fast food. My parents brought the rich flavors and aromas of South Indian food with them when they immigrated to Canada nearly forty years ago. I grew up loving spicy food. Living in Montreal and later Toronto during my medical training, my palette was exposed to the rich ethnic diversity that those cities' eateries offer. I enjoy exaggerated flavors: dark, bitter beer; strong coffee; fiery, hot burritos; well-aged cheese. Most fast food by comparison always seemed bland to me and I ate it rarely. After reading *Fast Food Nation*, I decided to avoid it completely.

I found myself at Pittsburgh Airport one morning without having had time to have breakfast and rushing to catch a flight to Kansas City. The airport was crowded as usual. Sharply dressed people queued up at every possible eatery hoping to be served as soon as possible. "Don't bother warming it up," I overhead one man telling a vendor selling calzones. Speed is key. Food at the airport needs to be *superfast*. Nearly everyone has a place to be at a precise time. As one of those people, I scanned the concourses for the shortest line. It's funny how people are willing to eat anything when they're hungry and in a rush. I lined up at a sandwich shop. The two servers moved numbingly slow. After ten minutes the line hadn't budged. Time was running out. I was either condemned to a tiny bag of pretzels on the plane or had to find another option quickly. One crowded outlet was serving customers at an incredible pace. Five lines of hungry travelers were ordering and receiving their meals in paper bags quickly. It was McDonald's, of course. I cast aside my vow to avoid that sort of fast food for the moment and bought a Big Mac value meal. I wasn't in line more than five minutes.

It smelled good even through the paper bag. The thick aroma of the crisp, slender, golden fries made my stomach grumble. I got to my gate only to find that my flight was delayed for thirty minutes. I pulled out the Big Mac. It was warm and felt good in my hands. After a few bites I started to think about what I was actually eating. Passages from *Fast Food Nation* came to mind. I lost my appetite quickly and put the bag aside. The pretzels on the plane would be fine, I thought.

Sitting immediately across from me was a family of Middle Eastern background. The father was eating a McDonald's hamburger. The mother, her head covered in a burka, was engrossed in a magazine. They had two beautiful little girls. One looked to be about five, the other, three. They sat facing each other on one of the soft bench-type seats. Between them was a red Supersize package of french fries. Mom had carefully laid down a couple of napkins upon which she poured out a few fries. She also squirted a couple of packages of ketchup in the center. When she saw what she was getting, the older girl clapped a few times. "We're getting fries. Yummy!" she told her little sister who didn't seem to quite grasp the significance of the event. With her tiny hand, the older girl reached down, grabbed a single fry, spun it around in the ketchup, and gently put it in her mouth. "Hmm . . . good." She then grabbed another ketchup-soaked fry and stuck it in her sister's mouth. Both girls started laughing. "Samira, look at me, I can eat three fries at a time!" The older girl did put three fries in her mouth, although I'm not sure she actually ate them. In any case, her little sister was delighted. With the utmost satisfaction, and giggling every couple of minutes, the two little girls consumed about a third of the french fries. Dad then offered both some of his soft drink, and they decided to give up on the fries and chase each other around the gate area. The innocence of childhood was so beautifully revealed by the humble french fry. Is fast food really that much fun?

THE RISE OF FAST FOOD

Fast-food outlets have become so much a part of the American land-scape that few people realize how many there actually are. I drove through California's wine country for the first time last year. The rolling hills are covered by tall, yellow grasses interrupted periodically by the lush dark green of vineyards. Some of the homes are really spectacular—white and pastel-colored mansions with Spanish tile roofs and elegant gardens. The countryside looks just like Tuscany or the south of France, except for one thing. Pull off the road in any small town and you'll see tall poles suspending the signs of America's favorite fast-food outlets. Outside of Napa, a giant sign for a fast-food chain is pinned up against the hills and the clear blue sky. Surely the view would be better without this intrusion, but for some reason the sign seemed like it belonged there.

In 1970 there were 30,000 fast-food outlets in the United States, or roughly one outlet for every 7,000 people. By 1980, this number had risen to 140,000, or one outlet per every 1,600 people. Today there are an estimated 247,115 outlets, or one per every 1,200 people.[2] The number of outlets continues to rise. To truly appreciate these numbers, consider the following: There are 170,700 gas stations, 127,000 super-markets, and just 118,000 public libraries in the United States.[3] The city of Los Angeles maintains and operates an impressive 124 public recreational centers throughout the city. McDonald's alone, however, has a bigger presence with more than 140 restaurants in Los Angeles.

The staggering number of fast-food restaurants is matched only by the amount of fast food that Americans consume. Fast-food sales total more than $130 billion annually, or roughly $440 for each man, woman, and child in the United States: 37% of adults and 42% of children eat fast food regularly. Consumption of fast food among children increased fivefold between the late 1970s and the mid-1990s.[4] The heaviest consumers are teens, who eat fast food an average of twice a week.[5] McDonald's even classifies its customers into how often they frequent its restaurants ever week.[6]

FAST FOOD AND OBESITY

There is a Wendy's down the street from my office at the University of Pittsburgh. It's an incredibly busy place that serves a large number of college students and faculty, healthcare workers, and school-children. I've learned a lot simply by watching what people order. I watched a heavyset boy around twelve or thirteen order the Classic Triple Cheese Combo. He upgraded his combo for thirty-nine cents to include Wendy's Biggie-size fries and a 32 oz. regular coke. That is a lot of food.

Before considering what makes up a Wendy's Supersized Classic Triple Cheese Combo, let's establish an important principle. The main thing to keep in mind about the fast food that children consume is its amount as measured in calories. Many Americans are obsessed with vitamins and other nutrients. I have many overweight and obese patients who insist on taking a daily multivitamin "for energy" but do little to balance the number of calories they consume and expend. It is true that fast food is poor in vitamins and nutrients. Still, there are nutrients in many of the other foods we consume. Vitamin deficiencies are extremely rare in the United States. With very few exceptions (e.g., vitamin D in some populations), the vitamin content of the foods children consume is far less important than how much they eat.

It is also true that fast food is often high in saturated fat and cholesterol, which increases the risk for heart disease. There is no question that children and adults should limit their consumption of fatty, cholesterol-laden foods. I believe nonetheless that calories should still be the primary focus.

According to *The Complete Book of Food Counts*, the Classic Triple with Cheese burger has an astonishing 810 calories; the Biggie french fries, 440 calories; and the 32 oz. Biggie drink, 244 calories. The total of nearly 1,500 calories is roughly equivalent to an entire fresh roasted chicken.[7] The Wendy's customer I observed is a growing adolescent boy who needs a recommended total of 2,000 to 2,500 calories per day. His single lunchtime meal at Wendy's, therefore, represents up to three-quarters of the calories he should be consuming all day. I hope he had a light dinner!

In a very entertaining way, *Supersize Me* confirms the relationship of fast food with poor health. The filmmaker (Morgan Spurlock) is a healthy, trim young man who decides to experiment by following a diet consisting of nothing but meals from McDonald's for a month. He "Supersizes" his meals whenever asked to by the sales clerk. The results are dramatic. Spurlock gains 25 lbs. His cholesterol level skyrockets. His liver function deteriorates. His mood and sex life suffer.

The film confirms that fast food in general, like soft drinks, has an unmistakable relationship to obesity. A recent survey revealed that compared to children who did not eat fast food, those who did eat fast food consumed 187 more calories per day. They also ate more fat and sugar and less fiber and milk and fewer fruits and vegetables.[8] The extra calories can be attributed to a couple of factors. The portion sizes of many fast foods, as in my example above, are huge. Fast foods are also full of fat and sugar, making even small portions "energy dense."

Let's consider the implications of an extra 187 calories per day. A child who eats 187 extra calories per day every day for a year will have consumed an extra 68,255 calories. A pound of fat (which is what those extra calories will be converted into) has approximately 4,000 calories. Those 68,255 calories will therefore be converted into an incredible seventeen extra pounds of fat! This is a simplified calculation. It doesn't take into account that growing children often need more energy, that there's a wide variation in how much physical activity children engage in, and that it's possible that children who eat fast food might need more energy for some unknown reason. These caveats aside, there is no question that children who eat fast food are going to weigh considerably more than those who do not. Not surprisingly, a study of young adults found that "heavy users" of fast-food outlets are 86% more likely to become obese over a fifteen-year period than young adults who eat fast food less than once per week.[9]

WHY CHILDREN LOVE FAST FOOD

Children love fast food for many reasons. Taste preferences develop very early and are determined to some extent by genetics. More important, early exposure to specific foods promotes acceptance later on in life. A recent study by J. A. Mennella showed that newborns who start with an unpalatable type of formula are more likely to accept it throughout infancy than newborns who start with a tastier formula and are later given the unpalatable formula.[10] A child fed turnips at a young age is more likely to have a taste for turnips later. In a world where fast food is everywhere and makes up a big part of the diet of adults, it isn't surprising that young children are exposed to fast food early and will find it tasty. Later, taste isn't the only thing that determines what children eat. A survey of high school students revealed that taste, followed by "getting a lot for the money," were the two most important factors that determined food choices.[11] Even adults rank taste and cost ahead of nutrition when choosing foods.[12]

Children (and adults for that matter) would never get to develop a taste for fast food unless they are drawn into fast-food outlets in the first place. Convenience is part of the attraction. Today's children lead busy lives. A parent shuttling children to soccer practice or a band rehearsal is likely to find that a quick stop at McDonald's or Burger King is an easy and inexpensive way to provide lunch or supper. The most important explanation for the love affair between kids and fast food, however, is, as in the case of soft drinks, marketing brilliance.

When I was four or five years old I remember watching a children's television show called *H. R. Pufnstuf.* In it, the lead character, Jimmy, and his talking flute, Freddie, are lured by an evil witch to a boat. A dragon named H. R. Pufnstuf rescues Jimmy and the flute and transports them to a magical "living" island, where everything, including books, candles, and the like, is alive and able to talk. I loved the show even though I was too young to fully appreciate the plot. I loved the colorful dragon and the catchy songs that Jimmy and Freddie would sing. Around the same time, I discovered what became another favorite television character. He, too, lived in a colorful, magical, musical land where everything seemed to come to life. His show would last only a few minutes but would appear often. I had a lot of trouble telling the difference between his show and *H. R. Pufnstuf.* His name was Ronald McDonald. His land was McDonaldland and his friends included the Hamburglar and Grimace, a talking purple milkshake. Ronald was a hero to me.

Ronald McDonald was based on Bozo, a clown character and children's entertainer who was popular from the 1940s to the 1960s.[13] The first Ronald was played by Willard Scott (now a weatherman). Interestingly, when McDonald's decided to make Ronald a national spokesman in 1966, Scott was fired for being too fat! Apparently McDonald's was keen to promote a fit, slim, youthful image of Ronald. McDonaldland, where Ronald joined his friends Hamburglar, Grimace, Mayor McCheese, and Sheriff BigMac, was invented in 1971. The Ronald McDonald character is more successful than any other advertising campaign in his ability to reach children. In *Super-*

size Me, several young children are shown pictures of President George Bush and Jesus Christ. None of them is able to name the pictures. All the kids, however, quickly identify Ronald McDonald. In fact, 96% of American children can identify Ronald McDonald. The only character with higher recognition among children is Santa Claus.[14]

The Ronald McDonald character is evolving and carefully designed to always appeal to children. For this reason, Ronald has recently come under fire from health and consumer advocates. He is certainly not the only reason children love fast food. After all, other fast-food outlets don't have a comparable spokesman. Children seem to love Wendy's too, though the late Dave Thomas, the founder and spokesman who appeared in many commercials, was certainly no childhood fantasy hero. Nevertheless, Ronald McDonald is an excellent example of how children perceive advertising, what appeals to them about it, and how it influences their behavior. These are issues worth understanding for you as a parent whose child is inevitably bombarded by advertising every day.

Television is by far the type of advertising that most influences children. Children exhibit different levels of vulnerability to advertising in general, and television advertising in particular, at different stages of their development. As noted earlier, young children don't "tune out" during commercials. The ability to distinguish between television commercials and regular programs surfaces at around age four or five.[15] Four- or five-year-olds, though they can identify commercials from regular programs, cannot really appreciate the difference. Their explanations are usually simplistic, such as "commercials are short."[16] Children begin to understand the purpose of advertising, that is, its "persuasive intent,"[17] by the age of seven or eight. Ninety-nine percent of ten- and eleven-year-olds understand the persuasive intent of commercials. Children eight and older also begin to recognize bias and deception in advertising. The number of children "liking all ads" decreases from 68.5% of first-graders to 55.9% of third-graders to 25.3% of fifth-graders.[18] As children get older, their own experience with advertised products shapes their views about advertising. They realize, for example, that toys seldom work in real life as well as they do in television commercials. Teenagers even develop cynical or antagonistic views about advertising.

Based on children's understanding of advertising at different ages, you would think that only the youngest children are vulnerable to its influence. It is true that children under eight are the most vulnerable. The skepticism that older children develop is known as a "cognitive defense"—a thought process based on knowledge and experience that makes them less likely to believe an advertiser's message entirely. Still, research has shown, unfortunately, that knowledge of advertising's persuasive intent and skepticism about its truthfulness does little to influence even older children's preference for advertised products.[19] In other words, knowing that an advertiser's main goal is to make money and that some products can be disappointing may make a child less vulnerable to advertising than one who can't distinguish between commercials and regular programming. But it doesn't make a child "immune" to advertising. This shouldn't be surprising. After all, adults are certainly persuaded by commercials.

Children's understanding of advertising at different ages explains why Ronald McDonald has been such a huge success. Ronald appeals to the youngest children. In his bright yellow outfit and red and white makeup, Ronald is an unmistakable presence on television. Ronald lives in a fun place and has fun friends. How could a young child think that going to Ronald's place (that is, McDonald's) could be anything but fun? McDonald's is, in fact, a fun place for children and not just because of the food. The restaurant chain is the largest operator of playgrounds, known as "Playlands," in the United States.[20]

Half of all the ads broadcast when television viewing among children is at its peak (e.g., Saturday morning) are for food.[21] More than a fifth of these are for restaurants. An analysis of food ads aimed at children revealed that taste and fun/excitement are the two most common primary themes in these commercials. Another theme is a so-called premium—a reward for eating the advertiser's food. The classic premium is the cereal box toy. For generations, children have been bugging their parents to purchase a brand of cereal just to get the little toy inside. Nutrition is among the least common primary themes in food ads aimed at children, though many breakfast cereal ads end with the ambiguous claim, "part of a balanced breakfast."

McDonald's not only has a great spokesman to reach children but also a menu that constantly changes to maximize appeal. The "Happy Meal" (its very title suggests fun) is the most successful children's menu item in restaurant history.[22] For more than twenty-five years the Happy Meal has always included McDonald's energy-dense food products in combination with an irresistible premium: graphics, puzzles, Teenie Beanie Babies, and a host of toys related to popular movies. Taste, convenience, and other factors aside, with its carefully crafted television advertising, its use of rewards to entice children, and its "Playlands," McDonald's is simply the king of "kid-appeal." This is why millions of children love it.

Chapter Four

Mesmerized by the Screen: Television and Other Media

One of my closest friends from medical school is a respected urologist at the Mayo Clinic. Greg is a disciplined, hardworking, "straight-laced," and likable Chinese American. On his twenty-fifth birthday, someone asked him, knowing full well that he wasn't a guy who had had a troubled youth, what he felt was his biggest mistake in life to that point. Greg responded, "I'd have to say dedicating myself so much to TV. It has literally zapped life out of me, and I don't just mean because of the time." He then went on to say that he could have used that lost time to learn how to play a musical instrument, a new sport, or a foreign language. I think my friend's comments were meaningful for a few reasons. First, many people would agree that watching television, especially for hours, is a waste of time. The alternatives, whether sports, music, reading, or other activities, are more constructive leisure activities since pursuing them leads to long-lasting self-improvement in ways that our society values. Most people are far more impressed by someone who has read all of Shakespeare's plays than by someone who has watched all the episodes of a particular TV show.

Time spent watching TV is time not spent doing something better. Greg's comments, however, indicate that lost time was not the only regret he had about watching so much TV. It "zapped a big chunk of life." Considering the fact that my friend is productive and happy, one could argue that watching a lot of TV has not really had much impact upon him. But I look at it from another perspective. Even someone like Greg feels that watching a lot of television as a child changed him profoundly. It *took something* away from him in addition to the time he lost. It's similar to the way people feel about substance abuse. There are successful people who have had to overcome addiction to drugs or alcohol and, of course, still regret their substance abuse because of how it affected their lives and the lives of those around them. Finally, a big portion of Greg's youth was *dedicated* to watching television. In this he certainly isn't alone. Television, for most people, isn't like going to the movies or playing golf. Golf is time-consuming and engrossing, but few people spend a large proportion of their lives golfing. Television is something people devote a significant portion of their lives to, whether It Involves watching or just thinking or talking about it. My friend Greg's rueful admission articulated the essence of television's impact on children, to which most of this chapter is devoted.

HOW MUCH TIME IN FRONT OF THE SCREEN?

I used to live adjacent to a lower-middle-class neighborhood in Pittsburgh called Morningside. Morningside is quiet and safe and has lots of children. There are several playgrounds and basketball courts and a baseball diamond. It's a nice neighborhood for a stroll on a warm summer evening. When I was a kid growing up in Halifax, Nova Scotia, playing outside in the summer until it got dark was considered normal. In Morningside today, the playgrounds are empty around 7 or 8 PM. Children are not out playing sports or riding bikes. Morningside's houses are built close together in an identical style, each with a big brick porch out front and a large window that looks in on a living room. Take a walk in the evening and you'll easily recognize the glow of a television from almost every house. Look closely and you'll see children of all ages sitting attentively in front of each TV. This is what millions of American kids do.

Ronald McDonald is not the reason why children watch so much television. The fact that children watch so much television is the reason Ronald McDonald is on the air.

Estimates of the number of hours children spend watching TV are astonishing. The average American child spends less time in school than he or she spends watching television.[1] In fact, more time is spent by children watching television than any other activity except sleeping. Children aged 2 to 17 watch an average of three and a half hours of TV a day. One in five kids watches thirty-five hours or more per week.[2] Television viewing starts at a very early age. Children as young as six to twelve months watch for one to two hours a day.[3] In other words, they learn to watch television before they can walk or talk. Viewing increases gradually during the preschool and early school years, peaks at around age 9, and declines thereafter.[4] Fifteen- to seventeen-year-olds watch about two and a half hours of television daily.[5] By the time the average American child reaches eighteen, he or she will have spent far more time watching television than talking to his or her parents.[6]

It is not hard to imagine that something that consumes so much of a child's time has a profound impact. A more fundamental question is, why do children watch so much television? There is no single reason. Very young children often don't make a conscious choice to watch TV. The TV is turned on to entertain them in the same way as their being handed a new toy. Television has served as a baby-sitter for more than fifty years. A survey of mothers in the 1950s found that many used TV as a pacifier and these mothers found that their children required less supervision and were less likely to misbehave while watching.[7] Paid baby-sitters, whether in a family home or a daycare center, certainly use television to keep children occupied. Interestingly, a more recent survey of American mothers showed that they were aware that many parents used television as a baby-sitter although they usually denied or were reluctant to admit that this type of baby-sitting took place in their own homes.[8] There is, in other words, a negative stigma attached to using television to keep children occupied.

As children get older they are able to make requests to watch television or can turn on the television themselves. Indeed 20% of two- to seven-year-olds, 46% of eight- to twelve-year-olds, and 56% of thirteen- to seventeen-year-olds have TVs in their bedrooms.[9] These are normally under their own control.

The reasons a child chooses to watch television are complex and varied and are worth understanding since they often pinpoint needs that are not being met in other ways.[10] Children use television for learning. This doesn't just refer to programs with a specific educational intent such as *Sesame Street*. Television is a source of advice to children. They may learn, for example, how to deal with problems with friends, parents, siblings, and the opposite sex. Disadvantaged children often use television to fulfill social or emotional needs that cannot be met within their own environments. A child doing poorly in school, whose own family is indifferent to the situation, for example, may learn how to cope from a television show featuring a child with a similar problem in a supportive family.

Television provides companionship in a couple of ways. When I was a child, television certainly brought my family together to share an entertainment experience. This still takes place, but far less often. Most children (especially the ones with TVs in their bedrooms) watch television alone. More important, television supplies children with a collection of fantasy friends. To young children, cartoon and other characters become people whom they can relate and look up to. Older children often find characters that serve as role models. Teenagers, especially those with few friends, frequently develop substitute friendships called "parasocial" relationships through television characters or the actors who play them. I have certainly heard many teenagers refer to characters from soap operas, reality TV programs, and other shows with a peculiar familiarity: "Did Amber do okay last night on *Survivor*?" Magazines that disclose the details of the personal lives of television stars are very popular among teens, especially girls.

Companionship and the familiarity with which children discuss television bring up another important reason for watching. Television is a great source of conversation. We have all been in awkward situations in which a small circle of people begin a discussion about a program or a movie they have recently seen or a book they have recently read, leaving out those who haven't shared the experience. The usefulness of television as a tool for socializing should not be underestimated. Several years ago I worked as an emergency room physician in a busy hospital in Toronto. I usually worked a night shift. On duty was a young, black security guard who had recently immigrated to Canada from the Caribbean. Most of the nurses on duty were middle-aged and had little in common with him. When not discussing work matters, this young man would talk to the nurses about nothing but popular daytime soap operas such as *All My Children*. They loved him for it. He, like the nurses, worked at night, slept during the morning, and awoke early in the afternoon to watch TV. This socializing value of television is even more important to children. Many children will actually selectively watch programs to make sure they are not left out of discussions among peers.[11]

Television provides an escape from the harsh realities of real life for both adults and children. Viewers can fantasize about a life that bears little resemblance to their own. Children who are frequently disciplined harshly or neglected by parents or have unhappy experiences in school are more likely to tune in to TV to escape. A study has shown that children who have recently been criticized or disciplined by an adult were more likely to watch a program in which children are praised or treated well than children who have not been recently criticized or disciplined.[12]

Escapism, companionship, and learning are important and often unrecognized reasons why children watch television. Children also watch for much more obvious reasons. Watching TV is simply a habit or a way to fill time. It provides entertainment and therefore arousal, or, depending on the type of program, relaxation. Think of the millions of kids seated in the back of minivans now equipped with DVD players. Watching a program helps pass the time on a long trip, enter-tains, or sometimes puts the young passengers to sleep.

TELEVISION AND HEALTH

When I was a kid, I was warned about sitting too close to the televi-sion because of the widely held belief that sitting too close could affect eyesight. Based on unscientific media reports, many mothers across America were also led to believe that TVs emitted significant amounts of radiation that could increase the risk of cancer among their children. These concerns about television were never based on good science and in any case have largely disappeared. The impact of television on children has since been rigorously studied. Blindness and radiation-induced cancer may be myths, but there is no doubt about it: Televi-sion has a significant impact on health.

OBESITY AND HEART HEALTH

An association between watching television and obesity among chil-dren has been observed for more than a decade. Some, however, still dispute the idea that television is linked to obesity.[13] The strongest evi-dence comes from a well-designed study published in the prestigious journal the *Lancet* in the summer of 2004.[14] Approximately one thou-sand individuals born in New Zealand in 1972 or 1973 were followed at regular intervals for twenty-six years. When the study participants were between the ages of five and eleven, their parents were asked how much television their children watched. Participants themselves were later asked how much they watched at ages 11, 15, and 21. The researchers explored the relationship between the number of hours of television watched as children and young adults, and body mass index, cardiovascular fitness, cholesterol level, smoking status, and blood pressure at age 26. The results were dramatic. Nearly half of twenty-six-year-olds who watched three or more hours of television a day were overweight compared to just 25% of those who watched less than an hour a day. The *Lancet* study also revealed that the more hours of television a child watched per day, the more likely he or she was to smoke, be unfit, and have high cholesterol as an adult. No significant relationship between television viewing and blood pressure was found. These are extremely important findings because, like obesity, high cholesterol, poor cardiovascular fitness, and smoking are risk factors for heart disease. Not only are heavy TV watchers fatter, they are at hugely increased risk of coronary heart disease, heart attacks, stroke, disease in the blood vessels of the limbs and neck, and the like.

The *Lancet* study found *associations* between TV viewing and cardiovascular health. In other words, it does not prove that TV viewing makes children fat. It can be argued that there is nothing particular about television that makes children fat and that children who are predisposed to becoming fat or are fat to begin with are more likely to watch television. In other words, it could be that TV watching doesn't cause fatness and that fatness causes TV watching. As I've discussed, children watch for many reasons. It isn't hard to imagine that children who are disadvantaged in some way adopt many self-destructive behaviors, including overeating and smoking, and turn on the TV to escape their troubles. The *Lancet* study did take this issue into account. It is known that socioeconomically disadvantaged children in rich countries are more likely to be obese. Children of obese parents are more likely to become obese. Children of smokers are more likely to take up smoking. The New Zealand researchers performed a statistical adjustment for socioeconomic status, parents' body mass index, and parental smoking. None of these factors could explain the association between childhood television viewing and health at age 26.

It is impossible to *prove* that television makes children fat. It simply isn't possible to conduct an experiment where different children are allowed (or forced) to watch different amounts of television, and then measure the impact on weight while controlling for all the other things that influence health. For similar reasons, identifying the negative health effects of smoking was challenging. Epidemiologists first uncovered an association between smoking and cancer nearly fifty years ago. For decades thereafter cigarette companies aggressively defended themselves by pointing out that epidemiological data did not constitute proof that smoking caused cancer. A comparably vigorous defense of children's TV viewing is unlikely. The soft drink and fast-food industries, despite evidence to the contrary, have continued to insist that their products are not harmful. There is no comparable lobby or group to defend children's TV watching. I've seen ads where trendy, healthy-looking teens pass up water, milk, or juice in favor of liquid candy. It would be hard to imagine an ad by the television industry showing a child choosing to watch TV instead of reading a book. The American people have accepted the idea that watching too much television is not a good thing. Fortunately, researchers no longer feel the need to confirm the association between television and health. They have moved forward to explore the actual potential mechanisms through which watching TV leads to childhood obesity.

There is nothing inherent about television that causes weight gain. If I took two seven-year-olds of exactly the same weight, asked one to read a children's book for an hour and the other to watch television for an hour, as you might imagine, afterward they would still weigh the same. Television causes weight gain by influencing other behaviors. A couple of these behaviors should be obvious by now. Children who watch TV spend less time being physically active and therefore burn fewer calories. Much of the advertising aimed at children is for unhealthy food. This advertising easily influences children. As a result, they pester their parents for fast food or other unhealthy products, or they make poor food choices themselves. Poor food choices lead to obesity. There is considerable evidence to support this chain of causation. Children who watch more television eat more high-fat foods and fast food, drink more soft drinks, and consume fewer vegetables.[15] In homes in which the television is on during meals, children consume more red meat, pizza, snack foods, and soda.[16]

A less obvious potential mechanism through which television

causes obesity is described in a paper by N. Stroebele and J. M. de Castro.[17] The eating habits of seventy-eight college students were compared on days in which they did and did not eat while watching television. The striking finding was that on days when students ate while watching television, their meal frequency increased. They ate nearly one full extra meal per day. This study should be interpreted cautiously. Once again it reports only an association. It is possible, for example, that college students have more free time on days when they eat in front of the TV and are also inclined to eat more often when they have free time. Whether the behaviors of college students are applicable to children is uncertain.

I will discuss the behavioral effects of TV watching on children in detail later, but one specific effect should be described now. In many cases, television acts as a stimulant for children. As mentioned, arousal is among the reasons children watch TV. A good proportion of children's viewing takes place in the evening or just before bedtime. It has been shown that television viewing before bedtime is linked to insomnia.[18] This shouldn't be surprising. Other stimulants cause insomnia and short sleeping hours in both adults and children. A cup of coffee just before bedtime is usually a bad idea. Japanese researchers have found a relationship between short sleeping hours in children and obesity.[19] Compared with children who got ten or more hours of sleep at night, children who got fewer than eight hours of sleep were nearly three times more likely to become obese.

There are several possible ways, yet to be thoroughly explored, that nighttime television viewing and consequent short sleeping hours could lead to obesity. Children who sleep less are typically tired during the day and may not be as physically active as children who sleep more. The secretion of growth hormone is lower in children who sleep less. Lower growth hormone levels are related to increased body fat. Cortisol, another hormone, is increased in people who sleep less. Higher levels of cortisol cause the accumulation of fat.

In summary, the association of obesity and television viewing among children is unquestionable. It isn't completely clear which way or combination of ways TV makes children fat. The influence of advertising and the substitution of TV for physical activity are almost certainly involved. The roles of stimulation by TV, insomnia, and hormonal changes on body weight are still being studied.

OTHER HEALTH EFFECTS

Obesity is only one effect of television. The impact of television on children, as my urologist friend implied, is far reaching. This book's subtitle refers not only to fitness and trimness but also to happiness. I think it is worthwhile for you to understand some of the other important ways in which television has an impact on a child's well-being.

Television and Reading

My practice in inner-city Pittsburgh is full of young children whom I often see for checkups. A checkup typically involves identifying health-related risks (such as obesity), providing health counseling to children and parents (such as telling a child to avoid smoking), administering immunizations, and obtaining routine laboratory tests. The purpose of a checkup is to make sure that a child is growing and developing normally. The kids are often very quiet and difficult to engage. When I need to discuss sensitive issues such as drugs, cigarettes, or sex, I, like most physicians, usually ask a child's parent or parents to leave the room. This sometimes helps the children to open up. Over the years I've used a few other tricks to make children feel more comfortable discussing not only sensitive matters but also sharing whatever else is on their minds. The best strategy is to find some common ground. This isn't easy. A physician in his thirties doesn't have a lot in common with a thirteen-year-old. The key is to know something, however small, about the culture in which the kid lives. Television is often the easiest cultural connection. I've never watched the *Power Rangers*, but asking a young child which Power Ranger is his favorite helped me score many points with kids a few years ago. I've seen very quiet young kids who normally make little eye contact come to life at the mere mention of *SpongeBob SquarePants*. Older kids are eager to discuss the latest videos by popular rap stars. Television not only serves as a source of conversation in these cases but also as a way of establishing a connection that makes it easier to talk about what many kids feel is the boring or uncomfortable subject of their own health.

All the children in my practice watch lots of television and enjoy talking about it. During a checkup, I also ask them about school. But I've found the need to ask very specific questions. "How are things going in school?" is usually met with no more than a terse "fine." I ask children to name their favorite subjects and teachers, the names of their closest friends, and to list their most recent grades. A child's life in school is undoubtedly an important window on his or her overall well-being. Most of the children tell me they are doing quite well in school. They proudly list the subjects in which they are getting As and Bs and then confess quietly to a couple of Cs and Ds that they insist "won't happen again." A couple of years ago I was shocked to hear that a significant percentage of American schoolchildren don't learn to read. I started asking children aged 9 and older to read as part of their checkups. I'll grab an easy-to-read pamphlet or children's book and ask each child to read a paragraph out loud and then explain its meaning. A few of the children do very well. They read in fluid, animated, articulate sentences, carefully placing emphasis on the right syllables. They provide nice concise summaries of each paragraph's meaning. Too many of the kids, however, do miserably. Some cannot read a word. Others can read the words with difficulty. Even those who get through an entire paragraph often cannot explain its meaning at all. Does television viewing offer an explanation?

A relationship between television viewing and reading ability has been reported for more than forty years. An important 1992 review found that television viewing and reading ability have an inverse relationship: the more television a child watches, the worse his or her ability to read.[20] The review also found that television viewing was inversely related to other measures of academic ability. This inverse relationship was strongest for children who watched more than three hours of TV a day, suggesting that three hours is a critical threshold beyond which academic performance declines sharply. How does TV viewing influence reading ability? The answer is more complicated than the fact that watching TV leaves children less time to read. C. Koolstra and T. van der Voort[21] found that children who frequently watched TV actually developed negative attitudes toward reading. Furthermore, TV watching diminishes a child's ability to concentrate while reading. In other words, watching a lot of television changes a child in some way that makes reading a less pleasant and more difficult experience.

Children who cannot read well have difficulty with oral and written expression. As they grow up, their job opportunities become limited. Their health may suffer, often as a result of poor understanding of health-related instructions. The implications of television's impact upon reading ability, therefore, are huge.

PSYCHOLOGICAL IMPACT

Television is not homogeneous. There is a staggering variety of programming available to children. Many programs are of educational value. Children's programs such as *Sesame Street* and *Reading Rainbow* are designed to improve, not hurt, a child's ability to read. Still, as noted earlier, television viewing among children has become a largely solitary experience. Despite recent efforts to control what children watch through ratings and the V-Chip, most children are exposed to the full spectrum of what television has to offer, including violent and frightening programs. As a consequence, television has a documented effect upon the psychological well-being of children. A survey of two thousand third-graders showed that as the number of hours of television viewing increased, so did the rates of anxiety, depression, and posttraumatic stress.[22] Frightening TV scenes have an immediate impact on kids: 62% of parents report that their children have at some point been scared that something they saw in a TV program or movie might happen to them.[23] A 1999 study revealed that children who had just seen a program depicting a drowning were less willing to go canoeing than children who hadn't.[24] The relationship of television to anxiety, stress, and depression among children is well established, but it has received far less attention than another important phenomenon: the impact of TV violence.

Violence on television and in other media has become so common that is taken for granted and sometimes not even recognized. Like most people of my generation, I watched the *Roadrunner* cartoon as a child, in which the Roadrunner's nemesis, Wile E. Coyote, tried repeatedly, though unsuccessfully, to destroy the Roadrunner with explosives, cannons, and falling rocks. Only after reflecting upon the show as an adult did I realize how violent it really was. Today's children are exposed to far, far worse and seem to have grown accustomed to seeing terrible violence. Beheadings of hostages are widely available on the Internet. You can actually buy these videos. Plenty of kids have seen them. A few schools even made the bizarre decision to show the video of the beheading of an American in class.

The television networks defend the amount of violence on television by claiming that it is simply a reflection of what goes on every day in America and around the world. Excluding the news, roughly 350 different television characters appear on prime-time television every night. An average of seven of them is murdered. Film critic Michael Medved pointed out that at that rate, the entire population of the United States would be killed in fifty days.[25] The idea that TV violence reflects ordinary life is preposterous.

By the time an American child finishes elementary school, she will have seen more than one hundred thousand acts of violence on TV, including more than eight thousand murders.[26] The impact of exposure to so much violence on TV upon the behavior of children has been studied for more than thirty years. Back in 1972 the US Surgeon General warned that "television violence, indeed, does have an adverse effect on certain members of society."[27]

The effect of TV violence is both immediate and long term. It has been shown repeatedly that boys and girls who view a violent program behave more aggressively immediately afterward toward other children and toward inanimate objects than children who do not view such a program.[28] More important, long-term studies have shown that the amount of TV violence a child views at age 8 is a predictor of violent criminal behavior at age 30.[29] Not every child who watches many violent programs, of course, grows up to be a criminal. Many factors predict criminality. The relationship between exposure to TV violence and aggressive behavior holds, however, even when one takes into account differences in social class, initial aggression, and intellectual ability. In fact, the association between exposure to TV violence and violent or aggressive behavior is nearly as strong as the association between smoking and lung cancer.[30]

OTHER MEDIA

TV screens are obviously not the only screens that capture children's attention these days. Among children, use of computers in general and the Internet in particular has exploded in recent years. As of late 2003, 35% of two- to five-year-olds and 60% of six- to eight-year-olds had access to the Internet.[31] Virtually all older children use the Internet. Children use computers for sending and receiving e-mails, playing games, word processing, browsing the World Wide Web, sending and receiving instant messages, and participating in chat rooms, as well as using them as an indispensable educational tool. Eighty percent of students aged 12 to 17 are given Internet assignments to be completed for school.[32]

The impact of computer use on children's health has yet to be fully explored. There are some key differences between computer use and watching television. The increased risk of obesity from sitting in front of a computer screen for hours is not likely to be too different than from sitting in front of a television, even though children surfing the

Web are not yet being constantly bombarded with ads for junk food. In contrast to TVs, however, computers are generally much more powerful educational tools. The Internet, for example, can be used as a tool to learn about weight loss or about maintaining a healthy weight. Also, computer use, unlike television, is an active or interactive activity. The psychological consequences are probably different and will become more apparent in the coming years. An early report found that the Internet promotes social isolation among heavy adult users, who spent less time talking to friends or family and attended fewer social events outside the home.[33]

Next to television, the electronic medium that has raised the greatest concern and received much attention, whether available on a computer or as a separate console, is video games. Video gaming has been around for a lot longer than surfing the Web.

A recent survey revealed that boys spend an average of 12.9 hours and girls an average of 4.9 hours per week playing video games. It has been shown repeatedly that children who spend lots of time playing video games perform worse in school.[34] The content of video games is an important determinant of school performance. If kids played only educational video games, their school performance may not suffer or may even improve.

Video game content has come under serious scrutiny for more than twenty years. When I was a young kid, playing video games meant visiting an "arcade" and feeding quarters into a machine featuring Space Invaders, Asteroids, or PacMan. The first home game consoles (e.g., Atari and Intellivision) became popular in the late 1970s and early 1980s. At that time a few computer enthusiasts also got the opportunity to play a limited selection of games on their home computers. Video game content was rarely called into question in the early days. Then, in 1983, came Custer's Revenge. This game featured a naked man in a cowboy hat whose objective was to perform sexual acts (which many critics described as rape) with a Native American woman tied to a pole. This was certainly not a product intended for children, but it did raise awareness of the whole issue of what can be sold as a video game and what children could be exposed to. Custer's Revenge was met by a ferocious public outcry. The company that created it promptly went bankrupt.

Today's video games, especially those intended for children, do not usually have such obvious pornographic themes. Explicit violence is the primary concern. Eighty-nine percent of all video games include some violent content. Fifty percent of video games include serious violent content (e.g., stabbing a video game character). Like violence on television, exposure to video game violence has an unmistakable relationship to highly aggressive behaviors. Adolescents who expose themselves to large amounts of video game violence are more hostile, more likely to get into arguments with teachers, and more likely to be involved in physical fights.[35] This once again raises the question of causality. Do video games make children more violent or are children who are violent to begin with choose to play violent video games? Both explanations are thought to be correct.[36] Children predisposed to aggressive or violent behavior often seek out violent video games. The content of games in turn may increase aggressiveness among them.

The relationship between video game playing and obesity, if any, is unclear. One study revealed that children who played moderate amounts of video games (roughly forty-five minutes a day) weighed more than those who played little or not at all. Strangely, children who played a lot of video games also weighed less than those who played moderately.[37] Maybe those who play a lot are so preoccupied by the screen that they forget to eat!

Chapter Five

Bodies Not in Motion: Physical Activity and Its Role in Weight Control

THE STORY OF THE PIMA INDIANS

Physical activity refers to the deliberate movements people make in a way that expends a significant amount of energy. It is widely believed that physical activity, just like what and how much people eat, plays a role in regulating body weight. Like many of the behaviors discussed in this book, diet and physical activity are closely related. Many inactive people have poor diets and vice versa. The tragic story of the Pima Indians of Arizona illustrates the impact of a poor diet and sedentary lifestyle, and offers some important lessons for all Americans about dealing with the problem of obesity.

Nathan Allen, a Pima Indian, provides an elegant and succinct history of his people.[1] The Pima Indians and their ancestors, the Huhukam, have lived along the banks of the Gila River in south central Arizona for thousands of years. The surrounding land is harsh desert. Like the people of the lower Nile in Africa, the Pima used their river to build a prosperous, agrarian society. They built an extensive canal system to irrigate crops of corn, beans, and squash. The Pima supplemented these staples with wild desert plants such as saguaro fruit, cholla buds, opuntia fruits, and a variety of wild nuts. The most important wild food was the mesquite bean. When crop harvests were poor, mesquite beans, usually ground into flour, provided sustenance.[2] Meat did not make up a significant part of the diet since large game was scarce in Pima territory. The river, however, was a good source of fish. Overall, the Pima had a varied and exotic diet. Harvesting crops and gathering wild foods must have been incredibly hard work. If you've ever seen a saguaro cactus in Arizona, you know that gathering its fruit must be no easy task. When the Spanish first encountered the Pima in 1694, they found a successful, self-reliant, and peaceful people.

The lives of the Pima remained virtually unchanged until the nineteenth century. The California Gold Rush brought prospectors through Pima territory in 1849. By this time, agricultural production among the Pima had become so successful that they began supplying the westward-bound prospectors with poultry, horses, mules, cattle, cotton, maize, and wheat. The Pima also sold enormous quantities of cotton, wheat, and corn to the Union army during the Civil War. Gradually, some gold seekers and others began to settle along the Gila River upstream from Pima territory. As their settlements grew, white settlers began diverting water from the river for their own crops. Downstream the Pima's crops began to fail. Already dependent to some extent on trade with white settlers and the government, the Pima began harvesting mesquite wood and selling it to railroads or to settlers as firewood. The desert landscape became changed forever.

By the time the Gila River Reservation was established as a home for the Pima in 1859, Pima society had already begun to crumble. A long period of battles over water ensued. Ultimately the Pima lost. Huge projects such as the Coolidge Dam were built with good intentions and designed to supply both the Pima and other farmers with enough water for farming. Unfortunately, much of the Pima's territory never recovered, so the Pima began abandoning agriculture altogether. Young Pima like Nathan Allen left the Gila River Reservation in search of work. After training as a welder in California and returning to the reservation, Allen wrote:

I found it totally different. The water situation had worsened, and the giant cottonwoods and mesquites along the earthen canals . . . had been ripped out. . . . The land seemed so barren and lifeless. There were fewer O'otham [Pima] farmers than when I had gone away to school. Large-scale Anglo farmers with modern machinery and financing capabilities were here leasing the lands once farmed by the landowners. . . . Somehow this just didn't seem like home. However, we had to move on. Although we were an agrarian people, we had to look for other means of revenue.[3]

To ease the suffering of the Pima, the government began a revenue-sharing scheme in the 1970s. The Pima tribe was given a specific amount of federal money to use for community and service projects. The Pima became completely dependent on this money. Pima territory became a welfare state. As the Pima descended into poverty, a host of other problems, including crime, drug abuse, and alcoholism, worsened. No longer able to grow food for themselves, the Pima's diet changed to inexpensive, highly processed, and calorie-dense foods such as packaged snacks and fast food. "Fry bread," a deep-fried combination of white flour and lard, became a new staple. The back-breaking labor that yielded such a rich and varied diet was replaced by boredom and television. The impact on health was so abrupt and dramatic that it has been the subject of intense research for nearly forty years. The Pima are among the most thoroughly studied people in the world.

For thousands of years the Pima were well adapted to surviving in the desert, where the availability of water is unpredictable. Abundant harvests were frequently followed by severe droughts. Unlike Americans with ancestors who lived in the rich, agricultural regions of Europe, the Pima have a genetic makeup that is perfect for a "feast or famine" environment. When such people no longer had to work hard to be well fed and had ready access to calorie-dense foods, the result was catastrophic.

The Pima are the most obese of all Americans. Young Pima adults have a body mass index that is seven to ten units higher than young adult Americans in general. This means, for example, that in comparison to the average American woman aged 20 to 29 who is 5'4" tall and weighs 142 lbs., the average young Pima woman of the same height weighs 183 to 200 lbs. Obesity puts the Pima at a very high risk of diabetes. In 1937 Elliott Joslin, founder of the renowned Joslin Diabetes Clinic, visited the Gila River Reservation and identified 21 cases of diabetes, a rate similar to that among all Americans. In 1954 there were 283 cases among a population of similar size. By 1965 the number had grown to approximately 500.[4] Today, roughly half of all Pima adults have diabetes, the highest prevalence in the entire world. Blindness, amputations, and kidney failure are extremely common. Type 2 diabetes has become common even among the young, affecting 8% of twenty- to twenty-four-year-olds and 3% of fifteen- to nineteen-year-olds.[5] The average Pima man has a life expectancy of just fifty-seven years,[6] lower than that of people in many third world countries.

Genetics puts the Pima at increased risk for obesity and diabetes, but it is the lifestyle of the Arizona Pima that has had a catastrophic impact. About three hundred miles south of the home of the Arizona Pima, high in the Sierra Madre Mountains of Mexico in a place called Maycoba, lives another group of Pima.[7] There are no significant genetic differences between the Arizona and Mexican Pima. The Mexican Pima, however, live in relative isolation. There is no electricity or running water. There are no laborsaving devices whatsoever. There is no television. The Mexican Pima essentially live the same way the Arizona Pima did a hundred years ago. Their diet consists primarily of beans, potatoes, corn, and small amounts of chicken. Nonmechanical farming and wood milling are primary occupations. The average Mexican Pima does between twenty-three and twenty-six hours of physically demanding labor a week. Only 6.4% of adults have diabetes. The average Mexican Pima adult weighs a remarkable 60 lbs. less than his or her Arizona counterpart.

PHYSICAL ACTIVITY, BODY WEIGHT, AND BODY FATNESS

The story of the Pima demonstrates the impact of a poor-quality diet *in combination with* a sedentary lifestyle upon a population susceptible to obesity. As we've seen throughout this book, there is no single factor responsible for the epidemic of obesity among America's children. There is evidence emerging that physical activity plays a role that is just as important as diet in maintaining a healthy weight. A recent study of the Amish supports this.

The Amish are a hardworking religious and ethnic group of European descent who live mostly in rural communities in Pennsylvania, Ohio, Indiana, Michigan, and southwestern Ontario, Canada. They are famous for preserving a culture that values self-sufficiency and shuns many conveniences most North Americans take for granted, including electricity and cars. Like the Mexican Pima, the Amish engage in an enormous amount of physically demanding labor. They also walk huge distances. Dr. David Bassett studied a group of "Old Order" (traditional) Amish in southwestern Ontario.[8] They spent much of their time performing physically demanding tasks. Dr. Bassett also asked each of ninety-eight Amish men and women to wear a device known as a pedometer for a week. (A pedometer counts the number of steps walked per day.) The Amish women walked an average of 14,196 steps a day or the equivalent of just over seven miles. The Amish men walked an average of 18,425 steps a day or roughly nine miles a day. One particularly energetic young man walked a remarkable 50,000 steps or twenty-five miles in a single day!

The Amish are committed to a very physically demanding lifestyle. The typical Amish diet, however, is nothing to rave about. A friend of mine who grew up in rural Pennsylvania among the Amish told me about one of the delicacies he enjoyed as a child. "Scrapple," also called "pawnhaus," is a mix of ground scraps of pork mixed with cornmeal mush that is baked into a loaf in a bread pan. The baked loaf is sliced and served with butter. Scrapple is typical of the Amish diet, which contains lots of high-fat, high-sugar foods including meat with gravy, eggs, and lots of pies and cakes. Does all that physical activity make up for an unhealthy diet? It certainly appears to do so in regard to obesity. Only 4% of the Amish that Bassett studied were obese.

It may seem obvious that physical inactivity leads to obesity. Indeed, it is easy to picture an overweight or obese child watching television or playing video games but difficult to picture the same child jogging or playing soccer. The relationship, nonetheless, is not that clear and depends partly on what criteria are used to identify obesity.

BMI is a simple and useful way to identify obesity, but it does not always correlate with how much fat a child actually has. Athletic children may have more muscle mass and therefore a higher BMI since they weigh more. Weight gain in puberty is expected and natural and also has an effect on BMI. For these reasons, some researchers use other measures of "body fatness" when studying children. In a recent European study, the activity levels of children were measured using a device called an accelerometer.[9] It measures the frequency, duration, and intensity of movements. Children wore the accelerometer at all times during the daytime for four days, except when bathing or swimming. This provided an accurate picture of their level of physical activity. The European researchers measured body fatness by measuring the thickness of skin folds over the arms, back, hips, and calves. As expected, the sum of the thicknesses of skin folds was inversely related to the level of physical activity. The least active children spent fewer than sixty minutes a day in moderate and vigorous physical activities and were the fattest. Children who spent more than two hours a day in such activities were the leanest. BMI and physical activity, however, were not related in such a significant way. Other evidence supports these results. Boys who play sports regularly, for example, have less body fat than those who do not.[10]

The finding that more physically active children are less likely to be obese brings up the old question of cause and effect once again. Does physical activity make children less obese, or does obesity make children less physically active? Strong evidence from studies designed specifically to determine if physical inactivity causes obesity in which children are placed in physical activity programs and the effects measured is surprisingly scarce. These types of studies are very challenging to conduct. Some physical training programs have been shown to modestly reduce body fat in children. All things considered, most experts today, based on the association of physical inactivity and obesity, accept the role of physical activity in controlling body weight among children.

ADDITIONAL BENEFITS OF PHYSICAL ACTIVITY

Physical inactivity promotes obesity and, as we've seen, obesity promotes insulin resistance, which in turn is closely related to a number of factors that increase the risk of cardiovascular disease. For this reason, physical inactivity can itself be considered a cardiovascular risk factor. A child who has one risk factor is likely to have several more. The presence of multiple cardiovascular risk factors in the same child is a phenomenon called "clustering." A recent study revealed that physically inactive children are more likely not only to have excess body fat but also to have the cardiovascular risk factors of high cholesterol and high blood pressure.[11] These are serious problems that can shorten the quality and length of a child's life. Being physically active, by contrast, reduces the number of risk factors. Diabetes, for example, is also a cardiovascular risk factor and can be prevented when children engage in vigorous physical activity.[12] There is as of yet no conclusive proof, however, that adults who were physically active only as children are protected against cardiovascular disease.[13] Many adults, despite physical activity during childhood, adopt unhealthy behaviors later on in life. This supports the need to remain physically active to maintain the health benefits.

Physical activity has a positive impact upon the mental health of children. Specifically, being physically active has been shown to improve self-esteem. Physically active children are less likely to suffer from mental health problems such as depression.[14]

Physical activity is also an effective way to reduce anxiety among children.[15] Proponents of physical activity often claim that school-based physical activities improve academic performance. Unfortunately, there isn't yet any good evidence to support this.

Weak bones (osteoporosis) are responsible for a significant number of fractures among the elderly. The strength of bones, measured as "peak bone mass," depends upon genetics, diet (as in the case of the impact of soft drinks, discussed earlier), and physical activity. The peak bone mass attained as an adult is largely determined over a short period of time during adolescence. Girls and boys accumulate bone mass at the highest rate at ages 12.5 and 13.5–14.0 respectively. Weight-bearing physical activities such as walking, jumping, and weight lifting have been shown to increase bone mass in children and teens.[16] Physically active children today are laying the foundation for healthy bones in young adulthood and beyond.

PATTERNS OF PHYSICAL ACTIVITY

Does a change in levels of physical activity help explain the epidemic of pediatric obesity? How physically active are today's kids? The answers to these questions are complex. It is useful to begin by distinguishing between two types of physical activities. *Organized* physical activity includes activity with an assembled group that has a coach, instructor, or leader. A children's soccer or baseball team is an example. *Free-time* physical activity refers to activity in which the child decides when, where, for how long, and with whom she participates. This is a deliberately broad definition that includes a large variety of activities. Riding a bike, for example, is a free-time physical activity, as is playing basketball with a group of friends (also known as "pickup" sports) after school or playing tag outdoors with a sibling. This distinction in types of activities is important since how much a child participates in each type depends on different factors.

Useful information on how active today's American children are comes from the Centers for Disease Control.[17] A recent survey of children aged 9 to 13 revealed that 38.5% participate in organized physical activities such as playing on sports teams; 77.4% participate in free-time physical activities. The most popular organized activities in this age group are baseball/softball, soccer, and basketball. The most popular free-time activities include riding bicycles and playing basketball. These numbers don't seem too bad since the majority of children are participating in some sort of physical activity. Looking at only these numbers, however, is deceiving. The patterns of physical activity among children depend greatly upon age, sex, and race.

One of my colleagues, Dr. Sue Kimm, published an influential study in the *New England Journal of Medicine* in 2002 that describes the patterns of physical activity among white and African American girls from age 9 or 10 to age 18 or 19.[18] More than two thousand girls were followed periodically over a ten-year period and their involvement in leisure-time physical activities was recorded using detailed questionnaires. These activities included both organized and free-time activities but excluded school gym classes, in which children can't usually opt out. Overall, physical activity declined by an astounding 83% between ages 9 or 10 and 18 or 19. By age 16 or 17, 56% of African American and 31% of white girls reported absolutely no leisure-time physical activity. By age 18 or 19 the vast majority of girls of both races were completely physically inactive apart from gym classes. Once girls leave or graduate from high school, they no longer have even the required gym classes to contribute to physical activity.

Dr. Kimm's study confirms several important findings that have been found in other studies. First, as children age, they become progressively more sedentary. This applies to both boys and girls though the decline in boys is not as steep as in girls. Second, the level of physical activity among girls is very low and much lower than that among boys. Even nine- and ten-year-old girls (the most active) are considerably less active than nine- and ten-year-old boys.[19] The gender differences in adolescence are huge. Finally, race is an important predictor of the level of physical activity. African American and Latino boys and girls are less physically active than their white counterparts.

Are today's children less active than previous generations? This is difficult to say. First, the differences between boys and girls and the decline in physical activity in adolescence have been observed for a long time. Second, participation in some organized physical activities is much higher than in the past. The number of boys and girls on sports teams has increased. The number of girls playing on soccer teams, for example, increased by 140% between 1990 and 2000.[20] By contrast, free-time physical activity has declined dramatically. Teenaged boys cycle only half the distance they did twenty years ago.[21] Walking was the most common way to get to school in the 1970s. Today most children get to school by bus or are driven by their parents. When I was a kid, it was popular to go to a soccer field, a basketball court, or an impromptu hockey rink on a frozen pond to play with whoever was available. It was usually the only chance that those of us without the talent to play on school teams got to play team sports. Such spontaneous or "pickup" play has never been popular among girls. It is now actually declining among boys. Overall, it is widely accepted that today's children are less physically active than previous generations.

What explains these patterns of physical activity among children? It is important for you to understand the reasons, because it will help you identify ways to encourage your child to be more physically active.

THE SPORTS PARADOX AND PHYSICAL ACTIVITY AMONG GIRLS AND BOYS

America is a country that takes sports seriously. Certain organized sports are attracting more boys and girls than ever before. In some cases, increased participation has extended into young adulthood. Among the most frequently cited successes in America is Title IX, the legislation enacted in 1972 to prohibit sex-based discrimination in higher education.[22] Still the impact of Title IX contrasts sharply with what is known about physical activity among girls.

Title IX is designed to provide men and women with equal opportunities to participate in competitive college sports. Since 1972 Title IX is responsible for a fourfold increase in the number of women participating on college sports teams. Every college receiving federal assistance is required to provide opportunities to participate on men's and women's sports teams in proportion to the number of its students that make up each sex. The number of men and women attending college is now roughly equal, so colleges are, according to the legislation, required to have as many places on women's teams as on men's teams or at least demonstrate a commitment to expanding opportunities for women. Title IX has become controversial because it has created some distortions. Many men are interested in playing on college sports teams, but colleges have in many cases been forced to cut positions on men's teams or eliminate men's teams such as wrestling altogether to provide balance according to sex. In some cases, in order to comply with Title IX and maintain their men's teams, colleges are recruiting young women with little interest in any sport to play on new women's teams. Women's rowing teams have popped up in colleges across the country. Ohio State University advertises for "tall athletic women, no experience necessary" to join its rowing team.[23] These distortions aside, most would agree that Title IX has had a significant impact upon athletic participation not only by young women but also by girls, who are seen as aspiring college athletes. In a recent article, Judith Rodin, the president of the University of Pennsylvania, declared:[24]

> Defenders of Title IX cheer the dramatic surge in women's teams and women's participation in intercollegiate sports. But the real beneficial impact of Title IX is not so much measured by the 157,000 women who play varsity sports in college, but rather felt on the youth sports scene, where schools and recreation programs afford girls and boys so many opportunities to play and excel in their chosen sports.

If so many women playing college sports are an inspiration to young girls, why as noted earlier are most girls finishing high school not physically active at all? This is the "sports paradox." Our society places a tremendous emphasis upon the traditional, competitive sports such as soccer, basketball, and baseball/softball. More girls and young women are participating in competitive sports at the highest levels. This has had little impact on the average, inactive teenaged girl who is unlikely to have the ability necessary to play competitively or the inclination to participate in the same sports recreationally or as "pickup" play.

Emphasizing high-level competitive sports has given some girls great opportunities, but if anything has alienated many others. The sports paradox applies to boys as well. The emphasis on high-level sports among girls pales in comparison to what boys have to deal with. People around the world have always been obsessed with success in men's sports. The obsession has sometimes reached fanatical extremes. In 1985 English and Italian soccer fans clashed in Belgium, leaving thirty-nine people dead. In 1992 a member of Colombia's national soccer team was murdered by an angry mob of his coun-trymen after he accidentally scored on his own goal. In western Penn-sylvania, where I live, football is an obsession. High school football regularly receives extensive coverage by local television stations. Col-lege football is the event around which weekends are planned. The biggest draw of all is the NFL's Steelers. Supermarkets, department stores, and even hospital emergency rooms are virtually empty during professional football games. Nearly everyone is either at home or at the stadium watching the Steelers.

Americans are now not only obsessed with sports played by grown men. Never before have American parents taken their sons' sports activities so seriously. Athletic prowess among boys, in many parts of the country, virtually guarantees popularity. Hardly anyone wants to hang out with the captain of the chess team. The quarterback of the football team, on the other hand, is usually among the most popular boys in school. Parents have become so obsessed with their sons' athletic accomplishments that psychiatrists have given this behavior a name: "achievement by proxy."[25] Fanatical and even violent behavior at sporting events is common. In 2000 a father who was angry about how his son's hockey coach was handling a practice beat the coach to death.[26] Boys used to play two or three different sports competitively on school teams. They are now, beginning as young as age 10, being encouraged to specialize in one sport in which they show the most promise and to play only the same sport year-round.[27] Does that sound like fun?

Despite the great opportunities girls and young women have to play competitive sports, and despite the great importance placed upon competitive sports among boys, overall physical activity today is lower than in the past and declines among both sexes as they get older. Our society has failed to make regular physical activity attractive for many children. This is the result of a failure to understand what motivates children to be physically active in the first place.

WHAT MOTIVATES CHILDREN TO BE PHYSICALLY ACTIVE?

What precisely motivates children to be physically active, or the "determinants of physical activity behavior," has been the subject of intense study for nearly twenty years. There are three broad categories of motivation.[28] First, children want to develop and demonstrate physical competence. This refers to athletic skills, physical fitness, and physical appearance. Second, children participate for enjoyment. Finally, children participate when provided with social support from adults and peers.

Children and Perceptions of Competence

The way in which children perceive themselves to be physically competent depends greatly upon their age and, beginning in adolescence, differs significantly between boys and girls. Young children judge their physical competence based upon successful completion of simple tasks, trying hard, and feedback from parents. A five-year-old playing soccer who successfully makes contact with the ball and aims it in approximately the right direction, for example, will feel competent, as would a child who tried to make contact with the ball unsuccessfully but was praised by his or her parent for the effort.

Children age 10 to 15 become much more competitive and gauge their competence based upon performance in relation to peers, as in *"I ran faster than everyone in the class today."* Winning becomes very important. Significant sex differences appear in the teen years as well. Teenaged boys are mostly concerned with competitive outcomes: *"We crushed the other team last night!"* Teenaged girls are more concerned with personal achievement goals: *"I was the MVP of the volleyball team three years in a row."* Teenaged girls also value feedback from adults and peers much more highly than boys. Significant differences in physical activity preferences by sex appear from age 10 to 14. Boys show a strong preference for games such as soccer and basketball. Girls prefer aesthetically and recreationally oriented activities such as dancing and skating.[29]

Creating an environment that helps boys and girl of any age feel competent is essential for engaging them in physical activity.

The Fun Factor

Children who enjoy organized or free-time physical activities are more likely to continue in them. Fun comes in different forms. Children enjoy the movement sensations of some physical activities. The exhilaration of skating across the ice at high speed or diving into a swimming pool is an important type of motivation. The social experience of participating in physical activity is also a significant source of fun. The camaraderie of a sports team, for example, is often the source of meaningful friendships. A 1986 study showed that one motivation for young gymnasts to continue participating in the sport was the fear of losing friends and letting down teammates and coaches by quitting.[30] Fun, however, has been shown consistently to be the most important determinant of physical activity behavior. It is simply not possible to engage a child in physical activity if he does not have a good time doing it.

Social Support from Adults and Peers

Social support for children involved in physical activity comes from parents, teachers, coaches, and other children. Parents play a vital role in motivating children through positive feedback and reinforcement: *"Even though you lost, I thought you played great, and you'll do better next time."* Boys typically receive more of this type of encouragement than girls. Sometimes overlooked is the importance of parents' own commitment to physical activity. A parent who is regularly physically active is more likely to inspire a commitment to physical activity in his children than one who is not.

Teachers and coaches usually provide feedback that is more objective and specific than parents. This takes two forms. Feedback can be informational or instructive, as in *"Let me show you how to hold the racket."* It can also be evaluative—either praise or criticism. Criticism of the right type is not necessarily a bad thing. A 1985 study by T. S. Horn[31] of thirteen- to fifteen-year-old female softball players revealed that players who were praised more often perceived themselves to be less competent than players who received more objective criticism. This is because the praise they received was often vague and given even after a mediocre performance, for example, *"Hey, nice job out there today."* The criticism, on the other hand, was much more specific and accompanied by suggestions for how to improve, for instance: *"I'm not happy with how you're throwing the ball to first base. Let's practice a few throws tomorrow."*

The influence of other children as a form of support is huge. Being physically competent virtually guarantees acceptance, support, and popularity among most children, for example, *"Hey, Tim. I'm playing on your line today. We're going to do great!"* Unfortunately, as discussed in chapter 2, children can be awfully cruel to each other. Being physically unskilled can make a child a target for ridicule and isolation.

Sadly, overweight and obese children are also often unskilled and thus suffer doubly as a result. There are so many stories of unspeakable cruelty. As noted in chapter 2, the scars that obese children bear from mistreatment can last a long time. I know of many adults who, though now fit and trim, were overweight or obese as children and still feel the pain and humiliation of having been taunted when they were young. I remember one case from my own childhood very well that illustrates the difficulties overweight and obese children face when they try to participate in organized physical activities. My seventh-grade gym class included a very overweight girl. On the first day of class she wore shorts and a T-shirt (which were required). She got teased for how she looked. For the second class, she came dressed in her street clothes and told the teacher she forgot her gym gear. He warned her to come properly dressed next time but allowed her to participate. We did some relay races that day. She did poorly. She got teased for that. For the third class, she conveniently forgot her gym clothes again. Visibly annoyed, the teacher told her that her behavior was unacceptable but still let her participate. We played soccer that day. Unable to keep up with the other kids, she got frustrated and spent most of the game on the sidelines. She got teased for that, too. I never saw her again.

BARRIERS TO PHYSICAL ACTIVITY

To be effective in engaging a child to be physically active, the activity needs to make children feel competent, it needs to be fun, and it needs to provide positive social support from adults and peers. Unfortunately, even activities that have these three characteristics may not be enough to engage some children, who face social and economic bar-

riers.[32] Some parents find it difficult to transport their kids to organized physical activities. The expense of participation, in the form of
registration or membership fees and sports equipment, is a significant
barrier for some families. Some families live in unsafe neighborhoods
and are therefore reluctant to let their children participate in organized
or free-time activities (e.g., riding bikes). Opportunities for physical
activities are limited in some parts of the country. These important
social and economic barriers are reported much more often by Latino
and African American families than by white families and may explain
the lower levels of physical activity among minority children. Overcoming these barriers has become a major priority for the Centers for
Disease Control. It will be an extremely valuable investment in the
future of America's children.

Chapter Six

The Family Meal
in the Twenty-first Century

THE EVOLVING FAMILY MEAL

T he childhood behaviors that can lead to obesity, which I've discussed so far, often take place out of parents' view. Children may drink soft drinks at home but are more likely to get them by feeding a few quarters into a machine or sticking a cup beneath a fountain dispenser at school. Children, especially teens, frequently eat at fast-food restaurants by themselves or with friends. I've already mentioned that television viewing these days is often a solitary experience. Physical activity, especially free-time activity, mostly involves other children in school facilities, backyards, and recreational centers. Parents are often not present. It would be easier, of course, to influence your child's behavior if you were always there to monitor soft drink consumption, for example. This would be impossible, not to mention overbearing. There is one place, however, where parents can have an unmistakable impact: the dinner table.

Family mealtime has undergone profound changes over the past fifty years. Television may contribute to making kids fat, but it offers a valuable glimpse of how the family meal has changed. In the late 1950s and 1960s the television show *Leave It to Beaver* featured the quintessential, almost perfect all-American family. Ward Cleaver was a hardworking accountant and dutiful father. June Cleaver was his devoted wife who seemed to spend all her time cooking, cleaning, or ironing. Theodore (Beaver) and Wally were the couple's clean-cut, well-behaved sons. With both pride and joy, June prepared classic American dishes like pot roast and mashed potatoes. At dinnertime, Beaver and Wally shared their experiences at school, including problems like poor report cards. The Cleavers were a family Americans admired.

The late 1960s and 1970s brought another almost perfect, albeit "blended," American family to the television screen. *The Brady Bunch* family featured six children. Dad was an architect. Mom stayed at home but was also a freelance writer, sculptor, and political activist. Unlike June Cleaver, Mrs. Brady was far too busy to cook dinner. Alice, their devoted housekeeper, took care of that. She must have been a good cook. *Alice's Brady Bunch Cookbook* has been popular for years. Brady family mealtime featured the same cohesion and openness as that at the Cleaver home. Ideal television families of the late 1970s and 1980s included the Bradfords (*Eight Is Enough*) and the Huxtables (*The Cosby Show*). These families also seemed to dine together although the family meal wasn't featured quite as prominently. Interestingly, *The Cosby Show*'s dad, Dr. Huxtable, took an interest in cooking once in a while. I'm not sure who prepared dinner for all ten Bradfords every night. It must have been quite a chore. America's favorite, though far from ideal, television family of the 1990s and today was and is *The Simpsons*. This satirical cartoon features a stay-at-home mom devoted to domestic chores, including cooking. Sadly, her family seems unappreciative of her efforts. Preferred family meals include trips to fast-food restaurants (e.g., Crusty Burger), outdoor barbecues, and steakhouses.

These television families may have little to do with twenty-first-century American family life. Older television families may not even have reflected American family life in their own time. After all, I'm pretty sure that real children in the 1950s caused more trouble than

Beaver and Wally. What is accurately portrayed is the importance of the daily evening meal. In the 1950s and 1960s dinner in a television family home was the highlight of the day. Preparing and consuming it brought joy. In the 1970s family dinner became less of a source of joy and more of an important social obligation. The task of preparing it was delegated to an outsider (at least for Alice, in *The Brady Bunch*). In the 1980s family dinner became less important. Teenaged television children could decide to dine out with friends. By the 1990s family dinner had become something occasionally to poke fun at. Cooking seemed a bit outdated. These trends parallel what has happened in our society.

Wally and Beaver always had dinner with their family. Today, only about one-third of all children and adolescents eat dinner with their families every day.[1] Children are less likely to attend family meals as they age. Fifty-five percent of twelve-year-olds eat dinner with their families daily compared to just 26% of seventeen-year-olds. Interestingly, children cite "not liking what's being served" as among the reasons they don't eat with their families.

The amount of time Americans spent cooking fell dramatically throughout the twentieth century.[2] June Cleaver spent hours making dinner, but her predecessors spent even more time in the kitchen. In the majority of households, women were and still are primarily responsible for preparing meals. Making dinner in 1900 was brutal work. Everything was made from scratch using sooty and inefficient coal and wood stoves. Iceboxes were available to keep foods cool but were nothing like today's modern refrigerators. Most food was purchased fresh, which meant several trips to the market or grocery each week. In 1900 the average American woman spent a remarkable forty-four hours a week cooking and cleaning up after meals. This was in addition to other household chores like laundry and dressing children. Preparing meals was more than a full-time job.

In the 1920s several innovations influenced the amount of time spent cooking. Electricity was widely available, so electric ranges, refrigerators, toasters, mixers, and other devices began appearing in American kitchens. Foods were now available in cans that could be stored for a long time. Many Americans had cars, which made the task of buying food much easier. In the mid-1920s, the average American woman spent about thirty hours a week preparing meals, a significant fall from 1900, but still a lot of time. During the Great Depression of the 1930s and during World War II, large numbers of women joined the workforce. American factories employed thousands of women during the war. By 1944, 35% of all women were employed, including 25% of married women. This, of course, had a huge impact on the time spent cooking. More innovative products appeared out of necessity.

The TV dinner, the grandfather of that great tradition of eating and watching TV at the same time, was introduced in 1954. Popular recipes were conceived around the same time not only for taste but also for convenience. These included casseroles—easy to make "hodgepodge" baked dishes. Weekly time spent on preparing meals dropped to twenty hours in the 1950s.

The 1960s and 1970s witnessed widespread use of important labor-saving devices, including the food processor and, most important of all, the microwave. Fast food, of course, became popular during this time period. Eating out was both practical and inexpensive. Weekly meal preparation time dropped to ten hours in 1975. The trends of using laborsaving devices and eating outside the home accelerated during the 1980s and 1990s as single-parent families became common and both men and women participated in the workforce in large numbers. In the late 1990s "home meal replacements," fully prepared but still fresh meals available from supermarkets and take-out restaurants, became hugely popular. Today, average daily meal preparation time is around twenty-five minutes (roughly three hours per week) and is expected to reach just fifteen minutes soon.[3] This isn't much time at all if you consider that it takes about five minutes to heat up a frozen calzone in a microwave. Basically, most days Americans no longer really cook.

Eating today, whether in or out of the home, is all about convenience. In addition to reducing meal preparation time by offering ready-cooked meals and designing foods specifically to be used in laborsaving devices (e.g., microwavable meals), the food industry is expanding the range of dining environments. A major focus of product development right now is the design of "handheld meals"—meals that fit conveniently in one's hand and can be eaten while walking or driving.[4] These superconvenient alternatives to sit-down meals will probably reduce both daily meal preparation time and the likelihood that families eat together even further. Already for some of today's children, the family meal isn't even a passing thought as they reach into the refrigerator for a pocket food and head quickly out the door.

Why does all this matter? First, when and how families eat together as well as the habits parents promote and the restrictions parents enforce upon their children all have a significant impact on children's weight and overall health. Second, as we'll see, the amount of time and effort spent preparing meals has had until very recently an impact upon the quality of what people eat. By quality, I mean the taste, freshness, quality of ingredients, and nutritional value of food.

THE BRITISH EXPERIENCE

Among Europeans, the British are not known for the quality of their cuisine. By contrast, famous and delicious dishes come from all corners of continental Europe. The Spanish have *paella*, the Italians have *agnolotti*, the Germans have *sauerbraten*, and the French have too many types of haute cuisine to mention. The French have been the undisputed champion gourmands of Europe for hundreds of years. Through much of the nineteenth and twentieth centuries, the British languished with their fish and chips. Until recently, British food had been bland, stale, and monotonous. A.V. Kirwan, the author of *Host and Guest*, remarked in 1864:

> The metropolis of London exceeds Paris in extent and population; it commands a greater supply of all articles of consumption, and contains a greater number and variety of markets, which are better supplied. We greatly surpass the French in mutton, we produce better

beef, lamb and pork and are immeasurably superior both in the quantity and quality of our fish, our venison, and our game, yet we cannot compare, as a nation, with the higher, the middle, or the lower classes in France, in the science of preparing our daily food.[5]

British food in the nineteenth century was awful. Yet it was not always that way. Medieval cooking in England was varied and tasty. The Venerable Bede (673–735), a monk and great scholar, on his deathbed carefully divided his greatest treasure among his closest friends: a handful of pepper. Spices were of great importance in English cooking for hundreds of years. In addition to adding flavor, spices, of course, also served as preservatives. The English sailed to India and Southeast Asia in search of pepper, among other treasures. Standard medieval English recipes reveal richness and attention to detail. Consider a popular recipe for what was known then as custard:

> Take veal and hammer it into little pieces in a pot, before washing it out. Then take clean water and boil powdered pepper, cinnamon, cloves, mace and saffron. Add plenty of wine, and boil the powdered veal in it. Cool the broth, take the white and yolk of eggs and strain them. Add them to the broth to stiffen it. Pour it into pie cases, along with chopped dates, ginger, and verjuice [fermented grape and apple juice], add it to the pie cases, and bake.[6]

Cinnamon, cloves, mace, saffron, chopped dates, and ginger? It all sounds very tasty—a far cry from fish and chips. So what happened? Academics have tried to answer this question for a long time. Many believe the Industrial Revolution was directly responsible for the precipitous decline in the quality of British food in the nineteenth century. The Industrial Revolution did help raise living standards and created a middle class. The middle class mimicked the habits of the aristocracy who rarely ventured into the kitchen. Cooking was regarded not only as unimportant but also as unsophisticated and uncultured. Hastily prepared dishes emerged. One nineteenth-century observer wrote:

a century ago the art of cookery was fashionable among English girls and Englishwomen . . . nowadays, piano mania and reception rooms are all that they think of; cookery is out of use, and only practiced by the lower orders.[7]

The decline in the importance of cooking paralleled a decline in the quality of food in Britain. Then, over a short period of time, there was what some call a food revolution. Large numbers of immigrants from the South Asian countries of India, Pakistan, and Bangladesh arrived in England in the 1950s and 1960s and brought with them the rich, spicy, though not necessarily healthy foods of their former homes. At first, this had little influence on British cuisine. The new foods were largely confined to ethnic enclaves into which the native-born British seldom ventured. The British gradually discovered the delicacies of the Indian subcontinent, and by the 1980s foods from India and neighboring countries had been integrated into the British diet.[8] There are now roughly seventy-five hundred Indian restaurants in Britain. Indian foods, as both raw ingredients and ready-made meals, are widely available in British supermarkets.

An even bigger contributor to the food revolution in Britain came from an unexpected source. Television cooking shows have been around for as long as television itself. American and Canadian cooking shows, until recently, have seemed to follow the same formula. A paunchy, middle-aged or elderly man or woman prepares a dish that requires many different ingredients and takes so long to make that the show's host presents previously made versions of the dish at different stages of preparation. The British, by contrast, have introduced the world to two very different celebrity cooks. Sexy Nigella Lawson prepares delicious simple recipes at lightning speed. The very hip and young Jamie Oliver has taken the world by storm by making cooking simple. Millions of Britons are huge fans of Nigella Lawson and Jamie Oliver. Celebrity cooks have not, nevertheless, reignited an interest in cooking among the British. The British spend less time cooking than Americans—averaging just thirteen minutes a day.[9] The revolution is the rediscovery by Britons not of cooking but of good food. Britain now has some of the best supermarkets in the world offering a fantastic variety of fresh produce and delicious ready-made meals based on ethnic recipes. Tesco, one of the largest supermarket chains, sells fifteen varieties of tomatoes in its shops. I counted just four varieties in a local supermarket in Pittsburgh. The British now enjoy food as good and as healthy as that available anywhere.

Britain offers some important lessons that I'll revisit later in this book. Changing economic times and demographics can reduce the attention paid to preparing meals and the importance of family dinner. Under these conditions, the quality of food served at home suffers. Exposure to good food creates consumer demand for it. The food industry responds accordingly, while still making things convenient. Convenience does not necessarily mean poor quality.

This revolution is taking place in North America as well. Retailers like Whole Foods offer convenience and quality. The Canadian President's Choice label's popularity is legendary in Canada and is the subject of a Harvard Business School review.[10] President's Choice offers an incredible variety of high-end meal replacements. Unfortunately, high-quality convenient foods have not yet enticed children back to the family dinner table.

HEALTHY EATING AND FAMILY DINNER

The preceding discussion should make it clear that I believe strongly that families should eat together. My reasons are not ideological. Many Americans lament the "breakdown of the American family" and reminisce about "happier" times when families like the Cleavers were more typical. The major television networks run public service messages (of questionable impact) hosted by celebrities encouraging parents to spend time with their kids or to discuss the negative consequences of taking illegal drugs. The setting for these messages is sometimes the family dinner table. This book is about the evidence in support of family meals—not about promoting or endorsing the somewhat intangible concept of "family values." I have many struggling inner-city single mothers in my own practice who would not likely be considered heroines of the family values movement. Yet many of these women, despite their financial problems and the frequent chaos in their lives, manage to include well-structured family dinners in their daily routine.

There is little good evidence linking the frequency of family dinner with obesity, but the family dinner is associated with improved diet quality among children. A study of more than fifteen thousand children of nurses revealed that children who ate dinner with their families every day consumed an average of 0.8 more servings of fruits and vegetables daily than children who ate family dinner never or on some days.[11] Furthermore, eating family dinner daily was associated with a much lower consumption of soft drinks and fried foods. These relationships are very strong. The more often a child eats dinner with his or her family, the more likely he or she is to have a better diet. As with other evidence, let's consider the issue of causation. Does family dinner lead to a better diet, or are children with better diets and healthier lifestyles for some reason more likely to have dinner with their families? The relationship between family dinner and diet quality holds after adjusting for a wide variety of other measures of healthy lifestyle, including television watching, body mass index, household incomes, and the presence of two parents in the home. In other words, other lifestyle factors cannot explain the fact that a child who eats with his family every day has a better diet.

There are different ways in which the family dinner is thought to improve diet quality. The first is obvious. Foods intended for dinner, whether made from scratch or home meal replacements, are generally much healthier than what children might otherwise eat. When children ask their parents "What's for dinner?" the response is unlikely to be potato chips and soft drinks. A less obvious mechanism is that eating dinner together encourages conversations about healthy eating. A survey of mothers and fathers who almost always ate dinner with their children revealed that nutrition was frequently the topic of conversation at the dinner table.[12] Family dinner, therefore, may be a means through which parents can encourage healthy eating practices among their children.

The family dinner appears to have other benefits. A recent survey of nearly five thousand adolescents in Minnesota revealed that adolescents who ate dinner with their families were less likely to use tobacco, alcohol, or marijuana, and were less likely to be performing poorly in school, have symptoms of depression, or express suicidal intent.[13] This shouldn't be too surprising if you've seen those public service announcements on TV that feature great parents who have great relationships with their children and ask their children about smoking and drugs. The Minnesota researchers, however, adjusted their results for "family connectedness"—a legitimate, accurate measure of how closely attached members of a family are to each other, based on questionnaires completed by the adolescents. The relationship between family dinner and the behaviors described above remained true. There is clearly something special about the family dinner that not only promotes good nutrition but also promotes healthy behaviors in general.

UNINTENDED EFFECTS OF PARENTS' FEEDING PRACTICES

In general, getting your children to have dinner with you as often as possible promotes good health. There are certain behaviors among parents, however, which, though well intentioned, actually have the opposite effect. Children are very vulnerable, and the way they respond to their parents' wishes and commands forms the basis of a complex science.

Young children (preschoolers) show a remarkable innate ability to regulate the amount of food they take in. In a 1993 study, children were given a regular diet that consisted of 10% of calories from ordinary fat for two days followed by a diet that included the 10% fat replaced by Olestra, a fat that is not absorbed and does not contribute energy to the diet.[14] The Olestra, therefore, removes 10% of the calories from the diet. The children involuntarily compensated for this lost 10% by eating more food (in the form of carbohydrates, etc.) to maintain a constant intake of calories over a two-day period. Unfortunately, as they grow older, children lose the ability to self-regulate their intake. How children are fed is believed to have a great deal to do with this.

Across America and around the world, children right now are probably making requests for food at inappropriate or unconventional times. I certainly did this as a child. Imagine a child who at 4:30 PM asks mom, "I'm hungry, can I have a cookie?" More often than not, the response is, "No, we're going to be having dinner in a little while." What effect does that have on the child? The child receives the message that it's the presence of food and not hunger that determines when to eat.[15] Most children at one time or another are told to finish what's in front of them. This "clean the plate" message also severs the natural link between hunger and food.

Severing the link between hunger and food interferes with a child's ability to self-regulate intake and can promote obesity. A 1987 study showed that when children were encouraged to focus upon feelings of hunger and fullness and were given meals with different amounts of energy, they were able to regulate their eating habits to maintain a constant energy intake. By contrast, when children were encouraged (not forced) to "clean the plate," they lost this ability to self-regulate and often took in more energy.[16]

Encouraging children to eat at times when they are not hungry is a common and harmful practice. Even worse are the practices of using food as a reward or restricting access to certain foods. Imagine a child who hears, "You can have ice cream if you finish your vegetables." What this actually does is increase the child's preference for ice cream and increase the child's dislike of vegetables.[17] In this case, good intentions have a negative effect on how the child thinks about food. The next time the child is offered ice cream, she is likely to enjoy it even more. Her mom and dad are likely to find it even harder to encourage her to finish the next serving of vegetables.

Parents often try to restrict access to foods that they know are unhealthy as a well-intentioned way to promote good health. These foods usually include sweets such as cookies, candy, and ice cream. Food restriction takes many forms. Foods can be put out of reach. When I was little, we had a big glass cookie jar high up on a shelf in the kitchen. I could see the cookies, but there was no way for me to get one. Food can also be allowed in limited amounts. A child may be given one scoop of ice cream or half a cupcake even though he knows that there is more available. Food can also be available only on special occasions. Ice cream, for example, could be served to children only when a family has company. Using food as a reward is another form of restriction. These practices are very common. In a study of 427 parents of preschoolers, 56% admitted that they frequently promised a sweet or other treat for eating a meal; 55% routinely withheld a special treat as punishment; and 48% rewarded good behavior with food.[18] The effects of food restriction have been studied extensively.

In one very elegant laboratory study from Pennsylvania State University,[19] a group of three- to five-year-old children was first asked to sample several different foods and to describe them as "yummy," "yucky," or "just okay." Based on their responses, two "okay" foods— apple bar cookies and peach bar cookies—were used for an interesting experiment. The children had equally neutral feelings about both types of fruit bar cookies and, when given samples of each, consumed them both in roughly equal amounts. For the next five weeks, apple bar cookies were restricted. Whenever the children came to the lab, they were given unlimited access to peach bar cookies. The apple bar cookies were kept in a large transparent jar and a bell was rung after which the children could reach into the jar to grab a cookie during a two-minute period. During the period of restriction, the children made many positive comments about the apple bar cookies and many more requests for them. They also made more attempts to get them, like grabbing and taking away the jar. Restricting access to a food that was initially considered nothing special made that food incredibly desirable.

It would be no major concern if food restriction resulted only in a few futile attempts by a child to get a desirable food or if it changed the attitude of a child toward a particular food. The problem is what happens when restricted foods do become available. In another Pennsylvania State University study, seventy-one three- to five-year-old children were given free access to ten different tasty snack foods, and the amount each child consumed of each snack food was carefully measured.[20] The mothers of the children were asked whether they restricted access to any of the foods. The degree of restriction was then compared to how much of the foods their children consumed. The results were striking and have important implications. The degree of restriction by mothers of a food was related closely to the amount consumed by girls, but not so closely to the amount consumed by boys. Boys did not significantly change the amount of each tasty snack food they ate when it was freely available, whether or not their mothers normally restricted it. Girls ate more of foods that were highly restricted than foods that were less restricted.

In general, trying to control when and how much of a particular food a child eats is now strongly believed to undermine a child's ability to develop self-control.[21] The lack of self-control explains the loss of the ability to self-regulate intake. The girls in this study opted to eat lots of a tasty food, simply because it was present, even when they weren't hungry.

The relationship between food restriction and poor eating habits is clear. The precise relationship between restriction and obesity is less obvious but believed to be significant. Not surprisingly, children's weight is related to food restriction. The heavier a child is, the greater the restriction by parents of sweets and other desirable foods. *Essentially, parents' misguided good intentions may actually be promoting rather than controlling obesity.* The mother of an obese girl concerned about her child's weight, for example, may restrict access to ice cream. When ice cream is available, the girl overeats it. Ice cream is very rich in calories and she is likely to gain weight, making her more obese. Her mother's response may be to impose even more restrictions, setting up a vicious circle of undermining self-control, overeating, and weight gain.

It isn't entirely clear why girls are affected more than boys by food restriction. It's possible that boys aren't too concerned about how their mothers or fathers restrict food. A more likely explanation is that parents monitor their daughters' intake more closely. Girls are more likely to face harsher restrictions than boys. Thinness among girls is emphasized constantly in our society. It has enormous social value. This may explain the degree to which girls' eating is restricted and the greater impact of restriction upon girls.

Among girls, food restriction may be partly responsible for more than just obesity. There are many risk factors and causes of the eating disorders bulimia and anorexia nervosa, both associated with an obsession with being thin and unhealthy behaviors such as bingeing and purging or excessive exercise. Restrictive feeding practices in childhood are believed to be among them.[22] Girls who have lost the ability to self-regulate based on hunger are going to be more susceptible to all kinds of environmental and social pressures. Their eating is prone to be "disordered" whether this results in being overweight or underweight.

In conclusion, restricting access to sweets and other unhealthy foods is not only ineffective in maintaining a healthy weight among children but may actually promote obesity. As you read this chapter, a clever thought may have come to mind. Would it make sense to restrict access to healthy foods among children to make them more desirable? Consider a household where asparagus is kept out of reach but in plain view of a child, or one in which spinach is offered only as a reward for behaving well! This is awfully hard to imagine. No one has yet studied the effect of restricting access to foods you would want to encourage your child to eat. There is no reason to think that such a strategy would work. Under any circumstances, as I've already discussed, exposing a child to new healthy foods at a young age is an effective way for him or her to develop a taste for them and to promote good eating habits in general.

Chapter Seven

The Truth about Diets, Programs, and Other Products

U p to now, this book might seem a bit gloomy. I've described an accelerating epidemic that has a huge current and future impact on America's children. The principal culprits are well entrenched in society and often supported by powerful interests. The soft drink and fast-food industries through their marketing clout have, for example, established millions of children and even the schools they attend as loyal customers. Helping your child achieve or maintain a healthy weight isn't easy given these forces and requires a commitment from you that is both intense and long lasting. The first important step is acquiring the knowledge you need. Now that you understand the importance of the problem of childhood obesity and its main causes, the next step is to learn how to solve it. Neither I, nor any other member of the health professionals community, has all the answers. The best I can do is identify the highest-quality information and translate it into practical recommendations for you and your child. Identifying the best information is a challenge because of the huge amount of misinformation that is out there.

THE WEIGHT-LOSS INDUSTRY

Americans are bombarded by more messages about weight than any other aspect of human health. Late-night infomercials, for example, in addition to handy kitchen appliances and get-rich-quick schemes, often feature miracle diets and strange-looking exercise equipment that promise to melt away the pounds with almost no effort. Adults and children interested in achieving or maintaining a healthy weight need to dig through a giant heap of misinformation to find out what really works. Like the industries that make people fat, the weight-loss industry is powerful and profitable. Americans spend approximately $40 billion annually on commercial weight-loss programs, related diet products and services, and diet-related media—an amount that is growing at a rate of 5.6% a year.[1] By contrast, just $4 billion is spent annually in the United States on cancer research.[2] The weight-loss industry spends millions on aggressive marketing of products and programs of questionable effectiveness.

Many people are desperate to lose weight, and there is a huge industry ready to take advantage of their desperation. This makes obesity an especially peculiar epidemic. People spend billions of dollars annually on products that make them fat. They then spend billions more to lose the fat. That money might not be so badly spent if it achieved a healthy equilibrium, meaning that people in the long run neither gained nor lost weight. Unfortunately, as I've discussed, both children and adults are getting heavier. This trend clearly benefits both the companies that promote obesity and those that promise to solve it. Eating an extra Big Mac a day for three months will cost you a total of about $225 and may cause you to gain 10 lbs. To lose the 10 lbs., you could enroll in a popular weight-loss program and if successful (and that's a big "if") expect to lose about 1 lb. per week. Ten weeks at such a program will cost you approximately $900. After a little over five months, you'd be more than $1,100 poorer, and the industries that have manipulated your weight would be that much richer.

There are several reputable weight-loss companies that have

helped many people, at least in the short term, achieve a healthy weight. The marketplace, unfortunately, is full of unscrupulous businesses that spread misinformation to lure people. Weight loss, of course, is not the only business in which the adage "buyer beware" is especially important. Buying a used car, for example, should also be approached cautiously. There are unique aspects of the weight-loss industry, however, that have allowed fraudulent programs and products to proliferate. First, weight loss is a very sensitive and deeply personal issue for many children and adults. As I've discussed, being thin carries an enormous social value in our society, especially for women. Fatness is associated with a lack of self-control and other character flaws. Think of all the things associated with thin women: beauty, youth, fitness, and energy. It goes way beyond that, however. The Duchess of Windsor once famously remarked, "You can never be too thin or too rich." Today, thinness and wealth often go hand in hand. Obesity disproportionately affects the poor. A lithe, well-groomed young woman is seen as upper class. Furthermore, thinness in women attracts the most successful men. I've had the opportunity, admittedly rarely, to attend a few dinners for Pittsburgh's leaders in healthcare, business, and education and their spouses. The only obese women there were among the servers and kitchen staff. What woman wouldn't want to be beautiful, rich, and fit into the upper echelons of society? The promise that thinness holds for a better life is what makes so many people desperate and extremely vulnerable to anyone who claims to offer thinness for a price.

Earlier I discussed the second important reason why bogus weight-loss products and services flourish. Obesity is an extremely difficult problem to solve and physicians have, for a variety of reasons, shown an inability or a reluctance to deal with it. This encourages people to look elsewhere for help. This phenomenon occurs with other problems as well. When I was a medical resident, I spent an afternoon a week for several months with a very likeable gastroenterologist in his clinic. He looked after patients with a number of different problems. His least favorite problem was irritable bowel syndrome, or IBS—a complex set of stomach and intestinal symptoms for which no obvious biological cause (such as an ulcer) can be found. Many physicians feel that psychological functioning plays a significant role in IBS. IBS is frustrating for physicians to deal with because patients experience genuine and sometimes disabling symptoms and yet there is no visible pathology to identify and treat. At that time the number of medications available for treatment was very limited. The gastroenterologist would try treating patients with diet modification and medications. The majority, unfortunately, would not improve. He would tell them, "In all honesty, I just can't help you. There's nothing I can do." Lots of his patients would then seek care from herbalists, chiropractors, and naturopaths. Others would spend a fortune on supplements that promised relief. I have no idea if any of the IBS patients found these alternatives helpful. I do know that an entire contingent of healers, some more credible than others, was ready and willing to provide its services. These healers all had one thing in common. They promised that what they offered would help. This is precisely what happens with obesity. The medical establishment has largely failed in providing effective care for overweight and obese people. The result is that patients are left to fend for themselves in a cesspool of sharks who promise weight loss and are ready to prey on their vulnerabilities and steal their money.

The weight-loss industry is so full of disingenuous hawkers that the Federal Trade Commission (FTC) launched a full-scale investigation into the problem, with a focus on weight-loss products. In September 2002 it released the results in a report titled *Weight-Loss Advertising: An Analysis of Current Trends*.[3] The report revealed that 40% of advertisements for weight-loss products included at least one false claim. An additional 15% of advertisements made claims that were likely to be false or were not adequately substantiated. Moreover, the FTC found that the number of misleading weight-loss advertisements had increased significantly over the preceding ten-year period. As the problem of obesity has increased, so has the problem of fraudulent claims of weight-loss products.

In November 2002 the FTC convened panels of scientific, industry, and media representatives to determine how best to address the problem of misleading advertising. The scientific panel reached a consensus about which popular weight-loss claims have no scientific basis. The industry panel was charged with the task of determining how best to regulate weight-loss ads to minimize deception. Not surprisingly, industry representatives favored self-regulation. The media panel also discussed the role of the media in spreading misleading weight-loss information. Media representatives cited the problem of the short time frame available to assess the quality of weight-loss ads before they are broadcast on television. The media panel did conclude that there is a need for a simple tool, based on the work of the scientific panel, which would help the media in making decisions about the truthfulness of weight-loss advertising.

Has the FTC done any good? As with many large initiatives of this type, the results are mixed. I still see blatantly fraudulent weight-loss claims all the time on television and in print media. On the other hand, consistent with the conclusion of its scientific panel, the FTC has produced a very useful guide designed for the media on how to assess weight-loss advertising. *Red Flag: Bogus Weight Loss Claims*[4] is also an extremely useful resource for ordinary people interested in weight loss. There are seven "red flags" that help media and consumers identify bogus advertising. A red flag is a claim that has absolutely no scientific basis.

The first red flag is a claim that consumers can lose two or more pounds per week without diet or exercise. Examples of such claims (created by the FTC to point out what to look for) include "No diet. No gyms" and "Fattacker: Attacks Fat!" The second red flag is a claim that significant weight loss can be achieved no matter what or how much someone eats. Such claims boast, "Eat all the foods you want and still lose weight. The pill does all the work!" The third red flag is a promise that weight loss will be permanent even when a customer stops using a product. Claims such as "Take it off and keep it off!" for products that are meant to be used temporarily fall into this category.

An ad for a product available without a prescription that promises to promote weight loss by blocking fat or calorie absorption is the fourth red flag. Claims of this type include statements such as "Brindall berries cause very rapid and substantial weight loss by reducing fat absorption by 76%." Red flag five includes claims that consumers can lose more than 3 lbs. per week for more than four weeks. These are the products that promise enormous amounts of weight loss: "How would you like to lose 30, 40, or 50 pounds? Now you can!" Red flag six is a promise that a weight-loss product will work for everyone. Consumers should watch for claims such as "Everyone in our study lost a substantial amount of weight." Finally, consumers should watch out for claims of patches, creams, wraps, earrings, and other products that are either worn or rubbed into the skin that promise weight loss. According to the FTC, no successful product of this type has ever been invented.

In addition to distributing warnings about bogus weight-loss claims, the FTC is now making a serious effort to impose penalties upon companies and individuals responsible for misleading advertising. Between June 2002 and January 2003 ads for a special weight-loss patch appeared as infomercials, on the Internet, and in magazines. Viewers and readers were told something like:

> Simply follow our system: Place a patch on your upper body. Then carry on with your everyday lifestyle. Every three days peel off the patch and watch as you take off the pounds. Replace with a new patch and drop more pounds. It's that easy.[5]

In infomercials this outrageous claim was accompanied by glowing testimonials from customers who had successfully lost weight using the patch. A testimonial by a woman named Tonya from Washington more accurately reflects customers' experiences with the patch:

> Boy do I feel stupid for believing in this product and also believing that I would actually get my money back with the "100% Satisfac-

tion." Please, please, do not fall for this "too good to be true" product. Even after I called to try and get my money back they charged me again for another shipment that I didn't even want. They are quick to take your money or charge your credit card but when you try and get a refund they will put you on hold forever and transfer you around until you finally just give up. I believe that it only works for those very few people that think it is going to work and convince themselves that it is going to be the answer to their weight problems.[6]

A man claiming to be a scientist provided explanations in commercials for how the patch works. His explanation included its ability to reduce fat cells and to produce and deliver its ingredients more efficiently than pills. The marketers of the patch were fined more than $1 million and prohibited from selling or marketing such products in the future.[7] Believe it or not, however, you can still buy this patch for $59.98 from a Web site that features the same outrageous claims as the infomercial.[8]

Weight-loss products often deliver far less than they promise. More relevant for the problem of childhood obesity are commercial weight-loss services. These include structured programs that incorporate dietary modification and other lifestyle changes. Like weight-loss products, the vast majority of commercial weight-loss programs target adults. Some reputable weight-loss companies have actually adopted restricted policies regarding enrollment of children in their programs. Weight Watchers Inc., for example, a highly reputable company, will not accept children under the age of ten and will accept children between the ages of ten and sixteen only if they have a physician's referral accompanied by a weight-loss goal and explicit parental consent.[9] Weight Watchers programs are designed for adults, and the company adopted this restrictive policy because of concerns that the programs would not be effective among children. Such candor in an industry full of charlatans deserves a great deal of respect.

Overall, the number of children enrolling in commercial weight-loss programs is very small and the rates of success are unclear. Nevertheless, learning how to evaluate the quality of commercial weight-loss programs is a useful skill because it helps you resist the temptation to invest in something that might not work and helps you educate your family, friends, and others interested in weight loss.

There are several excellent sources of information for consumers about how to choose a commercial weight-loss program, either for adults or for children. The Weight-Control Information Network of the National Institute of Diabetes and Digestive and Kidney Diseases (NIDDK) has a set of simple criteria for you to follow and questions you should ask.[10] A program should be safe and responsible. It should not include complete exclusion of certain food groups and should be designed to promote slow, steady weight loss of ½ lb. to 2 lbs. per week. Quality weight-loss programs also take into consideration cultural needs. In many cultures, there are restrictions on the consumption of meat or dairy products. A good program will provide culturally sensitive options in such cases. Programs should include a plan for increased physical activity in addition to dietary modification.

You should ask a number of questions before enrolling in a commercial program. What exactly the program consists of is crucial. Does it include individual counseling or group classes? Does it involve buying special foods or supplements? What activities does it offer? You should ask about the qualifications of the people who supervise the program. Are they nutritionists, physicians, exercise specialists, or other healthcare professionals? If not, what is their experience and expertise with weight loss? The risks of the program should be explicit. You should specifically ask about the risks of any supplements and/or drugs. You should ask whether a medical professional oversees the program and whether the program's supervisors will communicate with your own physician to make sure the program is right for you.

Questions about cost are especially important because this is an area in which a great deal of deception can take place. You should ask what is the cost of the program and if there are additional costs such as weekly attendance fees, costs of food and supplements, fees for follow-up visits, and fees for medical tests. Advertised initial enrollment costs can often be deceivingly low. Reading the fine print is essential.

Finally, you need to ask about the success of the program. The important question is, how much weight does the *average* participant lose and for how long, and how much of the initial weight loss is kept off? Commercial weight-loss programs are keen to promote their greatest success stories—the rare enrollee who loses a hundred pounds or more. The fine print beneath such success stories sometimes features a disclaimer of "Results not typical." Many people achieve short-term success in programs but regain the weight within a year. Specific questions about average long-term weight loss, therefore, will give you the best idea of the success of the program. It's a good idea to ask for references—people you can talk to who have enrolled in the program (besides their greatest success stories). If the directors of a commercial weight-loss program cannot answer these questions and the program doesn't meet basic quality criteria, you'd better look elsewhere.

DO COMMERCIAL PRODUCTS AND SERVICES WORK?

Knowing about fraudulent practices and the basic characteristics of reputable weight-loss programs is a good way to start becoming an informed consumer. Which commercial weight-loss products and services, if any, actually work? There is a large body of knowledge of what works and how it works published in the scientific literature (which I'll discuss shortly). Commercial products and services, however, rarely expose themselves to any serious scientific scrutiny. The result is that it is very difficult to determine whose sales pitch is legitimate. The red flags and basic criteria I discussed can help weed out obviously illegitimate players, but they are not helpful in evaluating the numerous other commercially popular weight-loss programs. The basic difficulty is that in the absence of objective scientific evaluations, we are generally left with only the information that the commercial enterprises wish to provide. The weight-loss industry, like any other industry, has its own commercial spin in providing information. I don't believe there's anything terribly wrong with that. A car dealer talking about his latest model is going to highlight its advantages over other cars and downplay its shortcomings. This is quite different from telling potential customers that his model uses virtually no gasoline, which is fraudulent. Commercial weight-loss programs also do this. If you really want to know how reliable a car is, you can ask other owners or, better yet, read a report based on the experiences of many owners. Similarly, the best way to find out about the effectiveness of commercial weight-loss programs is to ask the customers.

In 2002 the magazine *Consumers Reports* asked 32,213 adult dieters about their success in losing weight.[11] Roughly eight thousand, or 25%, lost at least 10% of their body weight and kept it off for at least a year, a widely used mark of success. Among these "successful losers" roughly half maintained their weight loss for five years or more. *Consumers Reports* calls these people "superlosers." According to the survey, therefore, about 75% of dieters were unsuccessful. What is more revealing is how the superlosers lost weight. Eighty-three percent of them lost weight entirely on their own, without the aid of a commercial product or service. The majority incorporated increased physical activity into their routine. Only 14% had ever enrolled in a commercial weight-loss program. By contrast, 26% of people who failed to lose weight had enrolled in a commercial program. Eighty-eight percent of superlosers did not use meal-replacement products. Only 6% of superlosers used dietary supplements or nonprescription weight-loss aids. The survey also revealed that the most effective organized weight-loss programs were sponsored by local hospitals and universities.

The *Consumers Reports* survey provides an important lesson. Significant, long-term weight loss can be achieved without the help of commercial products and services. In fact, adults who are successful in losing weight are more likely to lose weight on their own, rather than with the help of commercial programs. This doesn't mean that commercial weight-loss programs are useless. They do help some people. Through the *Consumer Reports* survey we saw, however, that the vast majority of adults interested in weight loss are better off trying to lose weight on their own, rather than investing time and money in a commercial program. This is even truer for children. As I said, commercial programs are designed for adults. It is much harder for children to follow a program's recommendations, even with a parent's help. If commercial programs are of limited usefulness to adults, they are probably completely useless in helping your child achieve a healthy weight. There is also evidence that some diet programs that are popular among adults may actually make obesity worse among children. Young children who are fed a low-carb diet (e.g., Atkins) or a low-fat diet, for example, are more likely to become obese teens than young children fed regular diets.[12]

Much of the weight-loss industry is prone to providing incomplete or exaggerated results. Information in the established medical literature is less likely to be commercially biased and is a good place to continue looking for what actually works. There are hundreds of studies of different diets, exercise programs, and other ways to change behavior. There is also a small but growing number of studies of new drugs for weight loss. (I'll discuss these in chapter 12.)

THE SYSTEMATIC REVIEW: SOME CLARITY IN THE CHAOS

One of the main objectives of the discipline of "evidence-based medicine" is to help physicians cope with the enormous amount of medical literature that is published regularly these days. The number is absolutely staggering. To put things in perspective, consider the following: in 1950 there were 87 articles published worldwide about obesity; in 1965, 244; in 1980, 1,100; in 1995, 1,525; and in 2003, 3,573. That's only about obesity. There are hundreds of thousands of articles about other topics published every year. Clearly it is impossible for any physician or other healthcare professional, no matter how diligent, to absorb such a huge volume of scientific information. Just to keep up with the literature on obesity, for example, would require reading nearly ten articles a day every day of the year.

The medical community has developed a number of tools to overcome this information overload. There are "screening" tools that help physicians find only the articles that are the most relevant for them and their patients. There are services through which someone else does the reading and then provides concise summaries of the relevant points of each article. The "systematic review" also developed in response to information overload. A systematic review is a type of study that seeks to answer a specific question by carefully examining previously published studies that address it. It attempts to synthesize the previous work in a way that allows physicians to draw conclusions. This is especially useful when two or more studies that address the same question reach different conclusions. Systematic reviews help clear up the chaos. They are relatively new to most physicians but actually have a long and interesting history.

I realize this is a book about "overnutrition," but allow me to describe a nutritional deficiency, the relevance of which will become clear in a moment. Scurvy is a disease caused by a deficiency of vitamin C. Virtually unheard of today, it was common right through the nineteenth century. The first symptoms include raised red spots on the skin around the hair follicles. The blood vessels that supply the hair follicles start to burst and the hairs no longer get the nourishment they need. Strands of hair fall out. A similar blight happens to teeth. Scurvy was especially common among sailors in the eighteenth and nineteenth centuries.

In 1747 a Scottish naval physician named James Lind decided to try out several different treatments for scurvy.[13] He took twelve sailors suffering from scurvy and divided them into six groups of two. Each group received one of the following treatments: vinegar; seawater; elixir vitriol (diluted sulfuric acid, something no one would drink today); a mixture of garlic, mustard seeds, and Balsam of Peru; cider;

and a combination of oranges and lemons. After observing the sailors for a period, Lind concluded that the oranges and lemons were the best treatment. Consuming citrus became a regular practice among British sailors. This is why they were called "limeys." Lind published his work in a paper titled *A Treatise of the Scurvy in Three Parts. Containing an Inquiry into the Nature, Causes and Cure of that Disease, Together with a Critical and Chronological View of what has been published on the subject.* It is this last part of the title that is especially important. Lind critically and chronologically, in other words "systematically," reviewed the existing literature on treatments for scurvy to that point. Lind wrote, "As it is no easy matter to root out prejudices . . . it became requisite to exhibit a full and impartial view of what has been hitherto published on the scurvy . . . by which the sources of these mistakes may be detected. Indeed, before the subject could be set in a clear and proper light, it was necessary to remove a great deal of rubbish." The systematic review was thus born.

The phenomenon of systematic reviews remained dormant until fairly recently. In the 1960s and 1970s British epidemiologist Archie Cochrane called for a large-scale, organized effort to develop systematic reviews in order to deal with the growing body of medical literature and the often-conflicting results of individual studies. In 1993 the Cochrane Collaboration was created in his honor. Its mission is to synthesize existing evidence into systematic reviews using very detailed methods. The collaboration includes physicians and other healthcare professionals from all over the world and has published hundreds of excellent systematic reviews. Earlier I told you I would translate the best evidence into practical recommendations that you and your child can use. To do that, I cannot read the more than fifty thousand articles written about obesity. I can rely upon high-quality systematic reviews that use rigorous criteria to determine what actually works in helping people lose weight, and then use that information to develop recommendations for you and your child.

There are two important systematic reviews that are extremely valuable in determining what works for obesity. In 2000 Danish

researchers C. Ayyad and T. Anderson published a systematic review
of all dietary treatments of obesity that appeared in the medical literature between 1931 and 1999.[14] They started by establishing strict
criteria for the studies they wished to review. To qualify for the systematic review, a study had to include treatment with diet alone or in
combination with any other therapy except for surgery. At least half
of the patients enrolled in the studies had to be followed for a period
of at least three years, regardless of the duration of the dietary program. Most important, Ayyad and Anderson established a strict definition of success. Studies had to show that patients kept off all the
weight they initially lost or at least 9 to 11 kg (20 to 24 lbs.) of the
initial weight loss over the three-year period. Ayyad and Anderson
studied treatments in adults only, but there are some important
lessons that are applicable to children.

You can imagine that if commercial weight-loss products or programs had to meet Ayyad and Anderson's criteria before being
advertised that you would hardly ever see an ad in the media. For
their systematic review, Ayyad and Anderson evaluated an incredible
898 previously published studies about diet therapy. Unfortunately,
only seventeen met their strict criteria. This says a lot about the state
of weight-loss research in the medical literature. The Danish
researchers put it bluntly: "The present literature study has revealed
the weak base for our knowledge on long-term effect of dietary treatment of obesity."[15]

Despite the lack of good-quality research, Ayyad and Anderson
were able to reach some important conclusions. First, the long-term
success rate of diets, according to their strict criteria, is a somewhat
dismal 15% (somewhat lower than the people surveyed by *Consumer
Reports*, but *Consumer Reports* used less strict criteria for success).
Diet programs are more effective, however, when they are combined
with one or more of active follow-up, group therapy, or behavior modification. *Active follow-up* simply refers to the opportunity for patients
to have contact with the weight-loss program after they have completed it. Many patients are left completely on their own after they

complete weight-loss programs. *Group therapy* refers to providing dieters with information or teaching them important skills in a group rather than an individual setting. *Behavior modification* is an approach to weight loss that encompasses many different techniques. Essentially, in addition to following a diet, people are taught to monitor and modify their behavior in a way that promotes weight loss. They may be asked, for example, to record when they get cravings for particular foods in a diary and then be taught how to deal with those cravings without giving in to them. Modifying behavior plays an even more important role in helping children lose weight and will be the focus of the upcoming chapters. Ayyad and Anderson's systematic review reveals that the best diet program is a very low-calorie diet (a difficult to sustain 300–600 calories a day) combined with teaching behavior modification techniques and active follow-up. This type of program is associated with a still modest 38% success rate. The lesson for dieters of all ages is clear—don't expect miracles.

The Cochrane Collaboration has published a systematic review titled "Interventions for Treating Obesity in Children."[16] This review considered not only diets but also all available therapies for treating childhood obesity described in the medical literature between 1985 and 2004. The Cochrane reviewers limited their systematic review to studies that followed children for a minimum of six months. To be included, a study had to compare children enrolled in a program to children not enrolled in the program. In such studies, children are usually randomly assigned to either be in the program or not. These types of studies are known as randomized controlled trials and offer the best-quality evidence. The Cochrane reviewers did not establish criteria for successful weight loss before starting their review.

Only eighteen studies that met the Cochrane criteria were found. These eighteen form the basis of the reviewers' conclusions. As in the systematic review of adult diet treatments, the Cochrane reviewers point out the lack of quality evidence that addresses the problem of childhood obesity. They also point out the discrepancy between how much emphasis childhood obesity receives and the seriousness of the problem: "While we agree that research in this area is difficult to conduct, this must be considered against a background which acknowledges that obesity is considered to be a global epidemic."[17]

What actually works for childhood obesity according to the Cochrane Collaboration? First, the broad category of techniques known as *behavior modification* has been shown to be consistently effective. Furthermore, behavior modification is more effective when the parents, rather than the child, are given the primary responsibility for the change. (This, of course, is the whole premise of this book.) Second, a technique known as *relaxation* is a promising approach to weight loss. Third, changing physical activity levels does work, but the evidence for *decreasing sedentary behaviors* (like watching television) is actually stronger than the evidence for increasing active behaviors like exercise. In the next two chapters I'll provide a close look at these effective techniques and advise you how to incorporate them into the daily life of your child and your family.

Chapter Eight

The Science of Changing Behavior and Its Role in Weight Control

THE NEED FOR A SCIENTIFIC APPROACH TO CHANGING BEHAVIOR

At this point in the book, the way to help your child achieve or maintain a healthy weight may seem fairly obvious: encourage your child to reduce or eliminate soft drinks and fast food from his diet; reduce his exposure to television; encourage him to exercise more; and make a commitment to have regular family meals. Sound easy? These goals are certainly very easy to define. It's often been said that any healthy person, no matter his or her starting level of physical fitness, can run a marathon with the right training. This is true. Successful marathoners include all sorts of people—even overweight office workers, senior citizens, and others who have set a goal that is personally important and have worked hard to attain it. The hard work includes drastic changes in one's health-related behavior.

As I'll discuss in chapter 12, medications, surgery, and other types of treatments may eventually be available for childhood obesity. For now, the safest and most effective way for a child to achieve or maintain a healthy weight is through changes in his lifestyle. One of the reasons so many weight-loss efforts are unsuccessful, among both adults and children, is because many people naively believe that changing behavior is easy. Physicians and other healthcare professionals often share this belief. This is one reason why we physicians often provide recommendations to eat right and be physically active in a casual, haphazard way: "Oh. Okay. Two things. First, I need you to come back in a week for me to check your shoulder again. Second, you need to eat healthier and lose weight. Okay?" The medical residents and students I teach often have complaints like, "I just don't understand why he doesn't diet and exercise more. It would really help his diabetes."

Most overweight and obese people want to be trim. Most smokers wish they could quit. Most alcoholics wish they could give up drinking. If changing behaviors that are destructive to our health were easy, everyone would be fit, trim, sober, and healthier. Changing behavior is clearly very difficult. I have been as guilty of taking a naive approach as anyone, as I'll explain next.

After completing some advanced medical training in 1997, in addition to my family practice, I started a job as director of community medicine for a hospital. My responsibilities included designing and directing health-related educational programs for people in different neighborhoods in Pittsburgh. Such programs are difficult to organize and very expensive to run since they require the participation of committed professionals with a high level of expertise. Within the scope of my role, I designed a course to be taught in five weekly one-hour classroom sessions called the Scientific Principles of Weight Control. The idea behind the course was that by teaching students how obesity is defined, the health consequences of obesity, basic principles of nutrition, and the importance of physical activity, students would be "empowered" to change their lifestyle and would therefore achieve or maintain a healthy weight. They would also empower other members of their families and even their communities. A contagion of weight-control empowerment would spread through Pittsburgh, and the city's obesity problem would be solved! An enthusiastic colleague and I approached the dean of the College of General Studies at the University of Pittsburgh to pitch the idea. The college caters to "nontraditional" students—generally adult high school graduates well beyond their college years who want a taste of college classes. The dean liked the idea for our course and hired us to teach it in the spring of 2000. The course was advertised in pamphlets all over the city. It cost only $49, which I believed was well within the budget of anyone interested in learning more about obesity.

On the first day, eight students showed up. One was a churlish elderly woman whose first question was, "Are you going to pay for my parking?" My refusal left her in a foul mood for the entire five weeks. My colleague and I administered a "pretest" to see how much our students knew about obesity at the beginning of the course and a "posttest" at the end of the course to measure how much they had learned. We also planned to weigh the students prior to the beginning of the course, at the end of the course, and six months later to see if we had had an impact. None of our eight students wished to be weighed. A couple of them dropped out halfway through (not the lady who thought parking was included). The remaining students struggled but ultimately came away able to answer questions such as "What is BMI?"

Our posttests revealed that the students did learn the material. Unfortunately, since they did not wish to be weighed, I have no idea whether the course had any other measurable impact. I doubt very much if anyone's weight was affected. On reflection, I consider the Scientific Principles of Weight Control course to be a flop. At the time, I knew a lot about the causes of and treatments for obesity, which was certainly essential. The fundamental reason the course flopped, however, was my failure at the time to understand the science of behavior change. I made intuitive assumptions about people's behavior based on my own attitudes and beliefs that were incorrect. Behavioral experts I spoke to afterward asked me difficult questions, which I was unable to answer: "What made you think that knowledge by itself would lead to a change in behavior?" "Was your idea for your course based on any well-established theory of behavior change?"

Psychologists and psychiatrists developed the science of understanding behavior and behavior change over the past fifty years. Within this science are several important theories and principles that apply to weight control. The science is very complicated and uses language that many people find hard to understand. My purpose here is not to overwhelm you with the details. I do believe that by understanding the basics of behavior change, you will be in a better position to help your child, and, more important, you will understand why things went wrong if and when your child doesn't at first meet significant goals. Health behavior change doesn't happen overnight. It is a long road with frustrating moments and setbacks along the way. For example, it takes an average of seven attempts for a smoker to finally quit for good.[1] Each failed attempt at quitting is a learning opportunity that sets the stage for the next attempt.

As noted at the close of the last chapter, behavior modification (especially as it relates to diet), decreasing sedentary activity, increasing physical activity, and the relatively new technique of muscle relaxation do work to help children achieve or maintain a healthy weight. Though the Cochrane review analyzed them separately, decreasing sedentary activity and increasing physical activity can be considered just two forms of behavior modification. The theories and principles I'll discuss in this chapter form the foundation of successful behavior modification programs for weight control.

EVOLUTION OF THE SCIENCE OF BEHAVIOR CHANGE

Early work in the science of behavior change was dominated by the idea that human behavior, like that of many animals, is controlled automatically and mechanically by triggers in the environment—the stimulus-response phenomenon. A couple of prominent scientists led the way in promoting this model of human behavior throughout much of the twentieth century. You may recall the work of Pavlov from your high school biology classes. Pavlov was the first to describe "classical conditioning" after experiments with dogs. The dogs would salivate whenever they could see or smell food. For a time, Pavlov rang a bell at the same time food was presented. Eventually, the dogs salivated automatically each time the bell was rung, even when food was not presented. They *learned* to associate the bell with food.

In the United States, B. F. Skinner was a pioneer in the science of behavior. Skinner developed the idea of "operant conditioning" by studying pigeons. He believed that behavior could be shaped by rewards. If he wanted a pigeon to turn to the left, for example, each time the pigeon turned even slightly to the left, Skinner would provide a food reward. The size of the reward increased with the size of the left turn. Eventually, the pigeon learned that left turns were in its best interest. Skinner believed that children also behaved this way and that everything humans do is based upon our experience with reward and punishment. He believed that the entire brain functioned in this simple, reflex manner. Essentially, Skinner didn't believe that the mind, as we think of it, exists.[2]

Pavlov's and Skinner's work, among others, formed the basis of *behavioral learning theory*: the idea that stimulus—responses—rather than thoughts, explain behavior. Behavioral learning theory can explain certain changes in behavior among children. A child is more likely to engage in a physical activity like playing outside, for example, if he receives a piece of candy as a reward.[3] In general, however, behavioral learning theory is now considered to be insufficient in itself to explain all aspects of health-related behavior.

Over the past thirty years, a number of additional theories, based on careful observations, that explain health-related human behavior have been advanced. Collectively these are known as "health behavior change models." Behavioral scientists and other researchers use them either to explain behavior or, more important, to design ways to influence behavior in a positive way. Let's say that a group of researchers wants to find an effective way to get teenage smokers to quit. They would start by selecting one or more health behavior change models and then design some type of program or tool, known as an *interven-*

tion, that fits the models. The type and content of the intervention would depend upon what the chosen models stipulate. For example, it could include a group class about the dangers of smoking or a booklet that would help teens keep track of when they get the urge to smoke. The health behavior change models that the researchers and others interested in changing the behavior of a group of people choose depends upon the problem they wish to tackle and the type of people they wish to reach (e.g., adults versus children).

Most modern health behavior change models recognize that behavior is more than the response to a stimulus. Some models are more successful than others in explaining behavior or as tools for behavior change. According to the *knowledge-attitude-behavior model*, health-related behavior changes come about slowly as one accumulates knowledge.[4] At a certain point, changes in attitude begin, and, as these accumulate, changes in behavior take place. For example, a smoker may gradually learn about the dangers of cigarettes, which would eventually influence his attitude toward smoking, which in turn would eventually lead him to quit. Unfortunately, increasing knowledge by itself has never been shown to be effective in promoting behavior change[5]—something I didn't realize when I designed the Scientific Principles of Weight Control.

According to the *health belief model*, behavior change depends upon one's beliefs about a particular behavior or illness.[6] There are five principal beliefs that make up the model: how serious one believes the problem to be; how susceptible one believes he is to the problem; how much benefit one believes he will get by changing behavior; the perceived barriers to behavior change; and how capable one believes he is to change the behavior. For instance, a woman with a strong family history of heart disease may be told by her physician to exercise regularly. She realizes that heart disease is serious and believes that she is at high risk. After receiving her doctor's advice and doing some reading, she believes that she can reduce her risk by exercising regularly. Unfortunately, she works long hours and has little time for formal exercise. She also doesn't feel comfortable working out in a gym in front of other people. She does feel comfortable and capable of getting up thirty minutes early every morning to take a walk, and she incorporates this into her routine.

The health belief model has been used to design successful interventions for adults. Children and adolescents often see themselves as invincible or immortal, so a model that emphasizes the seriousness of a condition or a child's susceptibility to it is not that useful in developing effective interventions. If I were to show a group of young obese children a video on diabetes that described how it is related to obesity and its serious complications, it would probably have little impact on the children's behavior. Similarly, you, as a parent, telling your child about the long-term dangers of obesity is not the best way to motivate him to eat better or exercise more.

According to the *stages of change* or *transtheoretical model,* behavior change takes place in five mental stages.[7] During *precontemplation*, one is not even thinking about changing health-related behavior. In *contemplation,* one is considering changing in the near future. In the *decision* stage, a plan for change is made. In the *action* stage, the plan is put into action. Finally, in the *maintenance* stage, the behavior change continues. This model takes into account the fact that not everyone is ready to change behavior. Many of my adult patients smoke. Some have never thought about quitting. Some tell me they plan to quit soon. Others are further along and are setting "quit dates," are in the process of quitting, or have quit and are fighting the temptation to restart. Programs for weight loss, based upon the stages of change model, have been designed with mixed results. The usefulness of this model to you as a parent in helping to change your child's behavior is yet to be determined.

Other health behavior change models include the interestingly named *theory of reasoned action* and the *theory of planned behavior.*[8] (A discussion of either of these is unnecessary.) The most useful model in explaining health-related behavior in regard to weight control is *social cognitive theory,* which was put forth by Dr. Albert Bandura in the 1970s. Bandura assumed that humans have the capacity to exercise control over the nature and quality of their lives, a characteristic known as "agency."[9] According to this model, health-related behavior can be explained as the result of an interaction between personal and environmental factors. Personal factors that determine behavior include *skills* (the ability to perform a behavior), *self-efficacy* (confidence that one can perform a behavior), and *outcome expectancies* (what one expects by performing the behavior). Important environmental factors include *modeling* (learning to perform a behavior by watching someone else) and *availability* (having the resources to perform a behavior). To illustrate these concepts, consider the example of an eleven-year-old girl and her involvement in organized sports. She has never played popular sports like basketball, volleyball, or soccer and never developed any basic sports skills. She also doesn't feel confident about playing any organized sports. The girl's parents both work and don't feel they have the time to drive their daughter to team practices and games. The girl, however, does ride a bicycle (availability) and is very confident about her ability to do so (self-efficacy). By riding her bicycle with her older sister, with whom she likes to keep up (modeling), she knows she will have fun (outcome expectancy). The older girl not only sets the pace but also rides regularly and encourages her younger sister to ride with her.

Without practical applications, behavior change models may seem like nothing more than "academic" ways to describe health-related behavior. Fortunately, behavioral scientists have been successful in using their understanding of health-related behavior based on models to develop successful ways of promoting behavior change. Their methods are known as *behavioral approaches* to specific health problems. For example, there are several behavioral approaches to quitting smoking that use the stages of change model.

The scientific literature on treatments for obesity in adults and children reveals that effective programs have certain common characteristics that together define a successful behavioral approach—that is, a successful approach to behavioral modification. The behavioral approach to obesity primarily makes use of behavioral learning theory and social cognitive theory. Aspects of the approach based on behavioral learning theory are more applicable to children than to adults. Now that you understand a little about the science of human behavior, you will be better able to appreciate why the strategies I'll describe next are likely to work.

THE BEHAVIORAL APPROACH TO OBESITY (BEHAVIORAL MODIFICATION)

In addition to its foundation in health belief models, the behavioral approach to obesity is based upon three intuitively obvious but important assumptions.[10] First, eating and exercise behaviors affect body weight. As you might imagine, this was proven long ago. Body weight is a function of energy balance. If you expend more energy than you take in, you will lose weight; if you take in more than you expend, you will gain weight. Second, eating and exercise patterns are learned behaviors and, like other learned behaviors, can be modified. This is also well grounded in science. Third, to make long-lasting changes in behavior, it is necessary to change the environment that influences behavior. This is consistent with the social cognitive theory that emphasizes the interaction of the "self" with the environment.

The first step in the behavioral approach is determining precisely what one hopes to achieve. *Goal setting* is an absolutely essential part of all behavioral programs. Goals should be realistic and customized to meet individual needs and preferences. Many behavioral programs include specific weight-loss goals such as a rate of loss of 1–2 lbs./week or a final weight-loss goal of 10% of initial body weight. It's also possible to establish behavioral goals such as cutting junk-food consumption in half or walking a total of twelve miles a week. Goals provide an essential motivation to continue healthy behaviors. Failure to meet goals is a useful gauge of success that provides an opportunity to reflect and learn from potential mistakes. This way future attempts at achieving a healthy weight are more likely to succeed.

The next vital step in the behavioral approach to obesity is fig-uring out precisely what behavior needs to be changed. This is achieved through detailed *self-monitoring*—recording every behavior that is related to weight. Following the behavioral approach requires, for example, writing down exactly everything that someone eats and drinks every day for several days. This diet record can then be reviewed to identify patterns that contribute to obesity. A diet record may reveal, for example, that an obese man has a healthy, normal diet most of the day, but he always gets hungry just before bedtime and has a big bowl of ice cream every night. A detailed record of physical activity may reveal that an obese forty-year-old woman exercises for an hour at a time, but only about once a week.

Once self-monitoring has revealed problem behaviors, the next step is to change the environment that controls the behaviors. The environmental influence on dietary and physical activity behaviors is best understood through what is known as the *A-B-C* model. Behavior is largely controlled by cues in the environment known as *antecedents* and by *consequences*, which reinforce the behavior and allow it to recur:

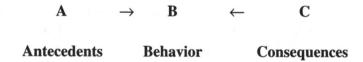

$$A \quad \rightarrow \quad B \quad \leftarrow \quad C$$

Antecedents   Behavior   Consequences

Consider the example of the nocturnal ice cream eater above. Feelings of hunger and knowledge that there is ice cream in the freezer are the antecedents that cause the behavior of indulging in ice cream. The man finds that the ice cream tastes good and fills him up. These con-sequences reinforce the behavior and explain why he eats ice cream every night.

Changing the environment in which behaviors take place can be accomplished by techniques known as *stimulus-control* strategies, which are especially useful for children. The antecedents are either eliminated or their influence is greatly reduced. In the case above, the ice cream serves as a powerful stimulus. Simply not having ice cream in the house changes the environment in a way that greatly reduces the chance that the behavior will take place. It is true that the man could drive to a late-night ice cream parlor to satisfy his craving, but a distant ice cream parlor is a far less powerful stimulus than ice cream in a freezer at home. Keep in mind that stimulus control is not the same as the unhealthy feeding practice of food restriction. A family that exercises stimulus control with respect to ice cream simply doesn't keep any at home to tempt children. Families that practice food restriction, on the other hand, do keep ice cream at home and make it available on a limited or "restricted" basis (e.g., as a reward for good behavior). Under such circumstances, the ice cream becomes a powerful stimulus.

Stimulus control is grounded in behavioral learning theory. *Cognitive restructuring* is a more "cerebral" strategy and deals not with a person's environment but with his thoughts. A person's thoughts frequently influence weight-related behaviors. This strategy aims to restructure those thoughts in a way that promotes a healthy weight. Imagine a woman who has had a long, hard day at work. She comes home thinking, "I've had a really tough day. My boss was so hard on me. I deserve to be treated better. I'm going to reward myself with a big piece of cheesecake." Cognitive restructuring teaches her to recognize that she is having these thoughts, to understand why they occur, and to replace them with thoughts that are more positive and compatible with good health. Something to this effect: "It sure was a difficult day and my boss was clearly not happy with my performance. This would be a good opportunity for me to take a long walk and to reflect upon what happened today, so that I can better understand my boss's expectations in the future." Of course, this is often much easier said than done. Cognitive restructuring is also more applicable to teens and adults than to young children.

Problem solving is another strategy that requires new ways of thinking and has been around for about thirty-five years. The technique is usually introduced to participants in a group setting. Individual participants are first taught to identify situations in which healthy eating or exercise is difficult. This is followed by an informal group "brainstorming" session to generate possible solutions based on the collective experience of the group's members. Individual participants try one solution and later evaluate its success. Many behavioral weight-control programs use group sessions. Problem solving allows them to individualize therapy by providing participants with skills that help them with their personal weight-control needs. Consider the following example: Stan, a fifty-year-old banker is trying to exercise regularly in the evening by jogging for twenty minutes around his neighborhood. He puts in long hours and finds that he is often too tired and unmotivated to do this, especially after dinner when his family demands his attention. His children often ask for help with homework. Stan's wife, who also puts in long hours, values the scarce family time available and would prefer that her husband not leave the house. As a result, Stan jogs infrequently and doesn't really feel that his exercise tolerance has improved at all. He is frustrated by his lack of progress. At a group session, participants in a behavioral weight-loss program offer several potential solutions: "Why don't you jog before work?" "How about jogging with your wife?" "How about buying a treadmill and putting it in your family room, where you would still be available for your wife and kids?" Stan doesn't feel the first two options would work. He is usually rushing to get ready for work and doesn't feel like he would have the time to exercise in the morning. Stan's wife is by no means unfit, but she doesn't feel ready to exercise with her husband. He buys a treadmill for $1,500. At first, he finds that he does exercise more often. He also feels that he is setting a good example for his kids, who see him exercising regularly. Unfortunately, within a couple of weeks, he becomes unmotivated again and the treadmill gets less and less use. He returns to the group to brainstorm about other solutions. The process continues until he finds an exercise routine that works for him. However, like cognitive restructuring, problem solving such as this is difficult for young children.

Relapse prevention is an integral part of most behavioral

approaches to weight loss. Lapsing or "slipping up" on occasion is a natural part of behavior change. People interested in weight loss are taught to identify and deal with situations in which they may slip. Consider a teen who regularly drinks a lot of soft drinks every day. With his parents' support, he decides to quit and switch to bottled water. Unfortunately, soft drinks are everywhere in his environment— at school, at his sports games, and at his friends' homes. On occasion, he does get a thirst for a regular soft drink and on one occasion has a can of regular cola. He feels terrible about this and wonders if he will really be able to quit for good. He discusses this lapse with his parents, who remind him that such slips are normal and help him to identify the circumstances in which he slipped and how he might cope with such circumstances in the future. He understands that the goal is to prevent him from reverting to his old pattern of drinking lots of soft drinks.

In summary, the behavioral approach to weight loss begins with defining precise goals based upon an individual's capabilities, needs, and preferences. Next, careful self-monitoring is used to identify problem behaviors. Strategies for changing these behaviors should include changes both to one's thinking and to one's environment. Stimulus control is used to change the environment and is especially useful in helping children achieve or maintain a healthy weight. Cognitive restructuring, problem solving, and relapse prevention are learned strategies that are especially useful for older children as well as adults.

WHAT MAKES SOME BEHAVIORAL PROGRAMS MORE SUCCESSFUL THAN OTHERS?

Though most behavioral weight-loss programs include the elements I've just described, not all are equally successful. Two key aspects of behavioral programs are very important in determining their success.[11] In 1974 the average behavioral weight loss program lasted eight weeks and the average participant lost about 8 lbs. By 1990 the average program lasted twenty-one weeks and the average participant lost close to 19 lbs. It has been shown repeatedly that the longer a behavioral weight-loss program is, the more weight that participants lose. Almost everyone regains weight after a program stops, but regular contact with a program helps maintain weight loss. Many behavioral programs based at universities, for example, invite participants who have finished a program to return periodically for support, counseling, and continuing education.

In addition to program length, social support has been shown to contribute to the success of behavioral programs. Individuals are likely to lose a bit more weight, for example, when a spouse joins a program with them.[12] Individuals who join weight-loss programs with a small group of friends have been shown to lose more weight than individuals who join alone.[13] The theory is that the social contact individuals receive from people close to them, who not only understand but also share their experience, provides support and motivation that increases the chance of success.

I just told you that the length of a behavioral weight-loss program and the degree of social support are two factors that determine success. It should be pretty obvious, therefore, who is in the best position to implement a behavioral program that will help your child achieve or maintain a healthy weight. Can you think of anyone who has more and longer contact with a child and can provide more support than mom and dad?

Chapter Nine

A Rational Approach to Achieving or Maintaining a Healthy Weight

At a recent dinner party someone asked me what I did for a living. I told him I am a physician and that my field of expertise is pediatric obesity. He responded, "So, what's your angle on that?" I asked him what he meant. "You know, what's your theory, your program, your fix?" Without getting into a long discussion about the different causes of obesity and the need for an evidence-based approach to the problem, I told him simply that there is no quick fix and that the same approach will not work with every child. My response might have seemed mundane. After all, as I told you in chapter 1, others are promoting much more exciting approaches such as eating according to blood type or feeding your child uncooked food. Such approaches are appealing for their simplicity, even when it's not clear that they work. People interested in losing weight desperately seek simple solutions to a complex problem. This doesn't make sense. Childhood obesity is the end result of a complicated interaction of genetics, family environments, and society. We've already seen the causes and consequences of obesity and the types of solutions that have the highest chance of working. Now that you have a greater understanding of the problem, something I feel is extremely important, it's time to consolidate what you've learned into practical recommendations. This book would not be useful without this chapter, nor would you be adequately prepared to help your child by reading *only* this chapter. What I offer is a set of recommendations with tips on how to carry them out, based on my interpretation of the scientific literature about childhood obesity.

Not every recommendation in this chapter applies to every child. If your child is very physically active, for example, increasing her level of physical activity should not be a priority. Furthermore, I wrote this book to be useful to parents of children of different ages. How you and your child use it will depend greatly on your child's age and level of maturity. As you might expect, the younger your child, the greater the responsibility you need to assume in carrying out the recommendations. A parent of a preschooler, for example, should be completely responsible for helping his child. Children age 6 to 12, depending on their level of maturity, can take a more active role in following the recommendations. Mom or dad or both, however, still needs to be firmly in charge. Young adolescents, age 13 to 15, should be equal partners in the effort to achieve or maintain a healthy weight. A parent of a four-teen-year-old should be asking questions like, "From what I've read, *we* need to cut down on your TV watching. What do you think about that and how do you think *we* can reach that goal?" Older adolescents, age 16 to 18, who are concerned about their weight, are typically independent and mature enough to find and carry out solutions to their problem on their own. If you are a parent of an older adolescent struggling with his weight, you can encourage him to simply read this book.

The recommendations in this chapter are based on what you've read up to this point. The best information on what works for childhood obesity comes from studies of well-organized programs often carried out in universities and hospitals. These settings are obviously quite different from the situation of a parent trying to help his child by reading and putting recommendations into practice. Nonetheless, there is no reason that what physicians, researchers, and others have learned over the past thirty years cannot be useful to a parent trying to help his child. After all, the importance of parental involvement in tackling childhood weight problems has been emphasized over and over again by researchers. Research may tell us what works, but, as I told you earlier, you, more than anyone else, are in the best position to help your child. I've simply panned through the science to find the "gold." What follows is my "angle." I've tried to make it practical, while not omitting important explanations. Goals have been bulleted and specific recommendations have been numbered. If you follow these recommendations, your child should be on his way to achieving or maintaining a healthy weight. It will not happen overnight. We each have one body to last a lifetime. Keeping that body in good working order requires a lifelong commitment. Achieving better health takes time. Furthermore, every child is different and I offer absolutely no guarantees of success in the form of weight loss in a certain time period, which would be irresponsible of me. I've numbered the recommendations. With the exception of setting goals and self-monitoring, they need not be carried out in sequence.

I. SETTING BROAD BEHAVIORAL GOALS

Based on what you've read, you probably already have a pretty good idea about what is contributing to your child's current or potential weight problem. In my experience, a bit of basic information goes a long way. I have a very overweight fourteen-year-old patient, for example, who is active in sports, never eats in fast-food restaurants, and limits the amount of television he watches. Unfortunately, you'll never see him without a plastic bottle of regular soda. He drinks soft drinks all day. He and his mother never realized how much this contributes to his daily intake and are now working to change what has become an entrenched habit. A general knowledge of your child's behavior should help you determine what needs to be changed.

The first step in helping your child achieve or maintain a healthy weight is to set broad goals based on your knowledge of your child's behavior. These goals can be refined as you gather more specific information. Many behavioral programs for adults establish specific weight-loss goals, such as a rate of weight loss of one pound per week. Specific weight-loss goals are not ideal for children for a couple of reasons. First, most children are still growing and maturing. Weight gain is natural as children get older, and keeping track of weight loss under those circumstances becomes complicated. An overweight thirteen-year-old girl in the midst of puberty may not achieve any weight loss at all despite pursuing a healthier lifestyle, because of the natural weight gain that takes place with maturity. Overemphasizing weight-loss goals might make her frustrated. Second, most would agree that the reason for children to maintain a healthy weight is to prevent the serious medical and psychological consequences of obesity throughout their lives. It is most appropriate, therefore, to set goals for lifelong changes in behavior. It is well accepted, for example, that children, young adults, middle-aged people, and seniors should all get some exercise on a regular basis. Setting a goal in childhood of engaging in some vigorous physical activity every day becomes a valuable precedent to set for the rest of one's life. This makes more sense than setting a goal for an adolescent of, for example, losing 20 lbs. in six months. Six months represent a tiny fraction of a person's lifespan.

A single set of broad behavioral goals applies to the majority of children struggling with their weight. Some goals may not apply at all to your child. At the outset, decide which broad goals do apply. There are some households where children do not watch television. Some overweight children are very physically active. Some kids don't eat junk food at all. In general, however, the most important broad goals include the following:

- Reducing or eliminating consumption of sweetened beverages (especially soft drinks)
- Reducing or eliminating consumption of "traditional" fast food (for example, french fries)
- Decreasing sedentary behaviors (especially television)

- Increasing physical activity
- Improving the environment of the family meal

II. SELF-MONITORING

I explained in the previous chapter that self-monitoring is a necessary early step in changing behavior. Positive changes are impossible unless you know precisely what needs to be changed. Self-monitoring should encompass dietary and other behaviors. Most professionally run behavioral programs make a significant effort to analyze the diets of their participants. Three methods are commonly used.[1] In some programs, participants are asked to keep a *dietary record* for a period of one or several days. This involves keeping track of everything one eats or drinks including the specific quantities. Nutritionists then analyze this information using sophisticated computer software. You can imagine that this isn't easy to do. Dietary records are sometimes so detailed and complicated that some participants in behavioral programs deliberately start eating foods that they know are easy to record, such as those with only one ingredient.

Twenty-four-hour dietary recall provides a snapshot of intake. Participants in behavioral programs are asked to reveal everything they have eaten over the past day. This, of course, doesn't necessarily provide an accurate picture since most people's diets vary day to day. *Food-frequency questionnaires* ask participants to record how often certain foods are consumed over a longer period, usually one month to a year. Unlike dietary records, which, when analyzed, provide a detailed picture of how much of specific nutrients one consumes, food-frequency questionnaires provide a more general idea of the quality of one's diet over time.

When completed properly, these three types of assessment tools provide an accurate picture of one's diet that can then be used to decide exactly what types of dietary changes need to take place. The problem is the amount of time, effort, and expense necessary to complete them and the expertise needed to analyze the results. This is why high-quality dietary self-monitoring is usually only part of organized programs that have many resources. It simply isn't practical for you and your child to complete a detailed dietary record, for example, enter the data into a software program, and analyze the results to identify problems. As an alternative, researchers continue to try to develop simpler, more practical tools, especially for specific populations such as children and minorities. As part of a program known as the Child and Adolescent Trial for Cardiovascular Health (CATCH), Texas researchers developed a relatively simple and accurate forty-item Food Checklist to measure fat and salt intake.[2] Even this is a bit complicated. To make things easy, I propose you use a simple questionnaire that focuses on the key "culprits" responsible for childhood obesity. Below is a questionnaire I developed for our center at the Children's Hospital of Pittsburgh:

Approximately how many servings of soft drinks (12 oz or 350 ml) does your child consume in a typical day?

___ (A) zero ___ (B) one or two
___ (C) three to five ___ (D) more than five

How often does your child eat fast food (e.g., Burger King or McDonald's) in a typical week?

___ (A) never ___ (B) once or twice
___ (C) three to five times ___ (D) more than five times

Approximately how much time does your child spend watching television, using a computer, or playing video games in a typical day?

___ (A) none to 1 hour ___(B) 1 to 2 hours ___ (C) 2 to 4 hours
___ (D) more than 4 hours

Apart from school gym classes, how often is your child physically active to the point of being "out of breath" in a typical week during the school year?

___ (A) never ___ (B) once or twice
___ (C) three to five times ___ (D) more than five times

In a typical week how often does your child have dinner with you and the rest of his or her family?

___ (A) five to seven times ___ (B) three to five times
___ (C) one to two times __ (D) never

There are no exact cutoffs for what constitutes unhealthy behavior. It is safe to assume, however, that As and Bs represent healthy behaviors and Cs and Ds unhealthy behaviors that require change.

The CATCH program also has an excellent checklist that includes other behaviors and specific instructions on how to set goals based on self-monitoring. You can access the checklist through: http://www.sph .uth.tmc.edu/catch/PDF_Files/healthy_habits%20_home.pdf.

A simple questionnaire like the one above will help you identify key problem behaviors. There are clearly other habits that contribute to obesity, such as eating too many potato chips. Based on your general impression of your child's behavior, you can modify an existing questionnaire or develop a new one. The objective is to have a precise idea of which behaviors and how much of them are contributing to the problem. Changing just a few behaviors can have a very big impact on your child's health.

III. REFINING BEHAVIORAL GOALS

Self-monitoring will reveal problem behaviors and set the stage for setting more specific goals. Specific goals should be customized to meet the needs of your child. They should also be realistic. To expect an overweight child who has never been physically active to participate in vigorous exercise for an hour a day, for example, is unreasonable. Goals should be attainable and can be refined as your child makes progress. This having been said, let me offer you some specific goals for the five problem behaviors I've emphasized throughout this book, based on recommendations, when available, from leading organizations. The goals for soft drink consumption and family meals are based on my experience and interpretation of the available evidence.

1. Soft Drinks

As I've stressed, soft drinks have no nutritional value and are contributing significantly to the epidemic of obesity among America's children. Recommendations in the scientific literature from physicians and nutritionists emphasize the need to eliminate soft drinks from schools. I think the term *eliminate* is key. There is simply no reason for your child to consume regular soft drinks.

Eliminate soft drinks from your child's diet.

This may be difficult to do depending upon your child's age and the amount he consumes. (I will discuss a few strategies later.)

2. Fast Food

In the film *Supersize Me*, Morgan Spurlock calls a number of nutritionists to ask them how frequently people should consume traditional fast food. Recommendations vary. One woman tells him that if he were stranded on a desert island with absolutely no other food sources then fast food might be something to consider! For obese children, it is of course best to eliminate traditional fast food (e.g., burgers, fries, chicken nuggets) completely from the diet. This may be hard to do, especially if fast food is part of your child's routine. There are no consistent recommendations in the scientific literature. The American Obesity Association recommends the following:[3]

Limit the frequency of fast-food eating to no more than once per week.

3. Television

Television is as much a part of American life as baseball, and *eliminating* it from your child's life is unrealistic. It would also deprive him of the quality programming for children that is available. The American Academy of Pediatrics has some very specific recommendations about television that I think every family should follow.[4]

No television at all for children under the age of two.

Limit television and video viewing to no more than two hours per day for children age 2 and up.

I would go further and include video games and the Internet in the two hours per day, with exceptions for using a computer for homework. Surfing the Web is an increasingly popular activity among children. Too much of it certainly isn't healthy.

Physical Activity

The Centers for Disease Control (CDC) promote different physical activity recommendations for adolescents and elementary school children.[5] The recommendations are ambitious and will not be easy for a very inactive child to reach. As I'll discuss, gradually working up to these goals over time is a good strategy.

All adolescents should be physically active daily, or nearly every day, as part of play, games, sports, work, transportation, recreation, physical education, or planned exercise, in the context of family, school, and community activities.

Adolescents should engage in three or more sessions per week of activities that last twenty minutes or more at a time and that require moderate to vigorous levels of exertion.

Elementary school–aged children should accumulate at least thirty to sixty minutes of age-appropriate and developmentally appropriate physical activity from a variety of activities on all, or most, days of the week.

An accumulation of more than sixty minutes, and up to several hours per day, of age-appropriate and developmentally appropriate activity is encouraged.

Some of the child's activity each day should be in periods lasting ten to fifteen minutes or more and include moderate to vigorous activity. This activity will typically be intermittent in nature, involving alternating moderate to vigorous activity with brief periods of rest and recovery.

Several definitions will help clarify these recommendations. "Accumulating" physical activity simply refers to the total amount of time spent daily being physically active. An elementary school child could meet the minimal recommendation by being physically active for twenty minutes three times a day. Physical activities are classified according to intensity as either moderate or vigorous.[6] Moderate-intensity activities include brisk walking, riding a bike slowly, dancing, or shooting baskets from one position. Vigorous-intensity activities include jogging or running, jumping rope, and most competitive sports.

5. Family Meals

There is no scientifically proven minimum number of family meals per week that will help your child achieve or maintain a healthy weight. As I've pointed out, we know that children who eat together with their families are less likely to become obese. The frequency of family meals obviously depends upon a variety of factors that may not be under your control. I urge you to make the best effort you can. I've also included some tips in this chapter on how to make the family meal setting healthier in general. All things considered, I believe the following recommendation is reasonable:

You and your child should eat together at home in a setting that promotes good nutrition habits at least four and preferably up to seven days a week.

IV. THE PROCESS

A child cannot reach the goals overnight. A reasonable strategy is to focus on a new goal every two weeks. For the first two weeks, for example, eliminating soft drinks could be the priority. If this is achieved in two weeks, you can move on to reducing the amount of television your child watches. There is no time limit for successful behavioral change. Some families may be able to reach behavioral goals within a couple of months; others may take a year or more. A parent and child who are actively trying to change behavior to promote a healthy weight should be applauded for their effort no matter how long the process takes.

Eliminating Soft Drinks

The process of eliminating soft drinks from your child's diet will be more or less difficult depending upon his age and how much he consumes. A preschooler does not make his own food choices. If you are giving your preschooler soft drinks, you need to stop immediately. Elementary school children may help themselves to soft drinks if they are available. Eliminating the presence of soft drinks as a stimulus in their environment is an important step. Make your home and other dining environments "soft drink free":

Get rid of any soft drink bottles or cans from your home as soon as possible.

Replace soft drinks in your refrigerator with healthier alternatives such as low-fat milk, water, or vegetable or fruit juices made from real fruit.

Serve as a model for your child by never ordering soft drinks with meals in restaurants or purchasing soft drinks from vending machines or convenience stores.

These basic environmental stimulus-control strategies will help the majority of kids give up soft drinks. A recent study from New Zealand[7] used classroom educational methods to discourage consumption of soft drinks. Children age 7 to11 were taught about what constitutes a balanced healthy diet and encouraged to drink water when thirsty. They also tasted fruit to learn about the sweetness of natural foods. They were shown a tooth immersed in cola and asked to evaluate its effect. Children heard a trendy song called "Ditch the Fizz," asking them to give up soft drinks and were also asked to produce their own song with a healthy message. This program was successful in reducing soft drink consumption, and, moreover, it offers a couple of lessons for parents.

An educational message about soft drinks can have a significant impact on children 7 and up. Tell your children that soft drinks are not part of a balanced, healthy diet, and that water is a better refreshment. Encourage them to try naturally sweetened foods such as fruits. This message may be used to promote cognitive restructuring among older children and adolescents. An adolescent who thinks "I sure could use a cola" can be taught that such thoughts lead to poor health in the long term. An adolescent should be taught to recognize when she is having such thoughts and that she may be thinking that way in response to thirst, a taste for something sweet, or the desire to reward herself. She should be told that thirst is best quenched with water, that a piece of fruit is a healthier and natural form of sweetness, and that she should choose some other sort of reward that may be a healthy food she likes or a healthy activity she enjoys.

A combination of creating a soft-drink-free environment at home, educating your child about healthier refreshments, and helping your older child recognize why she chooses soft drinks and how she can change her thinking should help her "ditch the fizz" for good. Even this single step will go a long way toward helping your child achieve or maintain a healthy weight.

Cutting Back on "Traditional" Fast Food

Limiting the intake of burgers, fried chicken, french fries, milkshakes, and other obesity-promoting staples of fast-food restaurants is crucial. Unlike soft drink consumption, I don't think it is absolutely necessary or practical to "eliminate" all fast food for a couple of reasons. First, many families rely on fast-food restaurants on occasion because they are convenient and inexpensive. A working couple with young children sometimes doesn't have the time or energy to prepare home-cooked meals. Giving up fast food completely may be unrealistic under such circumstances. Second, fast-food restaurants are beginning to respond to public concern over the nutritional value of their menus by offering healthier alternatives. In light of the need for convenience and the improving variety and nutritional value of fast-food offerings, the "once-a-week" recommendation of the American Obesity Association seems reasonable.

Parents purchase most meals for preadolescent children, and it is relatively straightforward for you to keep your preadolescent child away from traditional fast food more than once per week. Teens, on the other hand, often dine in fast-food restaurants by themselves. Many, of course, even work in such establishments. A fast-food restaurant may serve as a social gathering place for friends. This makes it harder for a teen to adhere to the "once-a-week" rule and to resist the smell of french fries or the taste of a hamburger. Parents need to make sure that teens understand the relationship between fast food and obesity. If and when a teen (or an adult for that matter) decides to visit a fast-food restaurant, he should bear in mind some practical tips to avoid overindulging in energy-dense foods:[8]

Control portion size. Choose a small sandwich, burger, or fries (e.g., a regular hamburger instead of a giant burger). "Supersizing" is being phased out of many restaurants, but always refuse this option if it is available.

Avoid high-calorie toppings such as mayonnaise.

Look for variety by choosing restaurants that offer more choices. Make a pledge to try all of the new healthy alternatives available in fast-food restaurants before choosing a traditional fast-food meal (e.g., McDonald's new salads with low-calorie dressing instead of a traditional fast-food meal).

Avoid soft drinks in fast-food restaurants. Milkshakes, which are also energy dense, should also be avoided. Choose water instead.

In addition to these tips, older teens may benefit from watching a video or DVD of *Supersize Me*.

Television

Reducing the amount of television your child watches is made difficult by the fact that television is such a big part of the lives of children. The TV Turnoff Network is a nonprofit organization that sponsors an annual "TV Turnoff" week and a school program called "More Reading, Less T.V." TV Turnoff Week is endorsed by the American Academy of Pediatrics, the American Medical Association, and the National Educational Association. The network also provides excellent tips on how to get your child to watch less television.[9] Most of these are classic stimulus-response strategies that rely upon strict enforcement of rules. Less potential television time means less watching.

The TV Turnoff Network recently conducted a survey of "TV-free" families that provides valuable information. Not surprisingly, TV-free families are well educated, spend lots of time together, and have children who excel academically and participate in sports and civic activities. Some of the statistics are truly astounding and worth reviewing.[10] Fifty-eight percent of school-age children in TV-free families are enrolled in "gifted" programs. More than half spend at least seven hours a week being physically active. Fifty-one percent get grades of mostly As in school. Forty-one percent of children old enough to read spent an hour or more reading every day. Children in TV-free homes spent more time with their siblings. Seventy percent of parents felt that their children got along better together because of no TV. If all this doesn't sound good enough, here's the clincher: only 7% of children in TV-free homes were ten or more pounds overweight. Most important for the purpose of this chapter, many surveyed parents who successfully eliminated TV from their homes did so by going "cold turkey." In other words, they simply stopped all TV watching completely. Children generally adjust within two weeks (though they may be hard to handle for a few days) and will learn to fill the extra time with more creative and healthier activities. This is what I recommend at first as well:

Forbid all television viewing in your home for a period of two weeks.

After this two-week period, you can reintroduce television to the limit of no more than two hours per day for children over age 2. The TV Turnoff Network offers tips on how to stick to this limit. I believe that some of these strategies are more sensible than others. The network recommends "hiding the remote control," for example, which I don't think would prevent a resourceful child from watching TV. The best strategies are the following:

If your child has one, remove the television from her bedroom immediately.

Keep the TV off during dinner. (This will help promote conversation.)

Don't use television for reward or punishment. Like food restriction, this may increase its value to your child. For example, "If you finish your homework early you can watch TV" or "Since you didn't wash the dishes like I asked, no TV for a week for you" can be counterproductive.

Cancel your cable subscription. Your television will lose some of its appeal, and you can use the money to buy reading material, educational software, etc.

Explain rules to your child in a positive way. Instead of saying, "You've reached your limit for TV for today and can't watch anymore," say, "Let's turn off the TV and read a story together."

Don't use TV as a baby-sitter. As an alternative, try involving your child in household chores or encourage him to play in a safe area outside.

These tips should apply to all types of electronic media, including videos, video games, and computers (except for school purposes).

Physical Activity

The CDC's recommendations for physical activity will take time for the majority of inactive children to attain. If your child is completely inactive, I suggest you take things slow. "Developmentally appropriate" activities for preschoolers include playing hide-and-seek or tag with a parent or sibling, riding a tricycle, or playing in an outdoor playground. Once your child reaches school age, in order to meet the

CDC guidelines, both free-time (or *habitual*) and organized physical activities should be incorporated into his routine. In other words, it is simply not good enough for a twelve-year-old to go swimming three days a week for half an hour and to be sedentary on other days. There are a few things I believe you should definitely do:

Begin a program of daily walks with your child.

The benefits of a daily walking program should be obvious. Both you and your child will reap the health benefits. Many parents complain that they don't get the chance to spend much time with their children or that they aren't sure what's going on in their children's lives. Walking with your child gives you the time to have conversations you might otherwise not have. An evening walk, for example, is an ideal time for you to find out about your child's day at school.

A pedometer is a simple device that clips on to your waistband and records the number of steps you take. Pedometers come in a number of colorful designs and are available from many retail stores (such as Wal-Mart and Target) for as little as $5. Purchase one for you and one for your child. Teach your child how to use it and encourage her to wear it daily. A total of ten thousand steps (the equivalent of five miles) a day is widely recommended as the amount of habitual activity needed to control weight.[11] For a parent or child unaccustomed to being physically active, this is far too ambitious an initial daily target even though it includes walking around the house, at school, and elsewhere. Start with a daily walk of one thousand steps and work up gradually to about twenty-five hundred steps (1½ miles). Make your walks an even more social experience by taking routes that pass by the homes of your child's friends or by a field where a sporting event is taking place. Notwithstanding the amount of time you have, take as many breaks as you like.

There may be several important barriers to a daily walking program over which you may not have much control. Finding the time for a half-hour walk may not be easy for many families. Walking early in the morning before school and work requires a great deal of motivation on the part of you and your child. Evening walks may interfere with time for preparing meals, doing homework, and the like. Some families live in neighborhoods where safety is a concern because of lack of sidewalks or crime. As always, do the best you can, realizing that the long-term benefits of a walking program outweigh the inconvenience.

Teach your child how to increase physical activity in his daily routine.

There are simple ways to incorporate increased physically activity into the things your child normally does that will help him achieve or maintain a healthy weight.[12] Here are a few important tips.

Tell your child to use stairs instead of elevators or escalators whenever reasonable and possible.

When arriving somewhere by car with your child, park at the far end of the parking lot and walk to where you need to be (e.g., at a shopping mall).

Assuming safety is not too great a concern, refuse to drive your child very short distances (e.g., to a friend's house). Tell him to ride his bike or walk instead.

If your child is old enough, insist that he help with chores that burn a lot of energy such as mowing the lawn, raking leaves, or shoveling snow.

Regular walking prevents weight gain. Children should also incorporate more intense, organized physical activities into their routines. In addition to walking, organized physical activity programs are available all over America, even in some of the most economically challenged neighborhoods. The key to engaging your child in an organized program is finding one that is appropriate for him. Ask yourself two questions: Will my child enjoy this activity enough to look forward to participating in it whenever he can? Will my child be able to sustain his participation throughout childhood, into adolescence, and possibly even in adulthood? As I told you earlier, children are motivated to participate in physical activities to demonstrate physical competence, to feel enjoyment, and to receive social support from adults and peers. This first motivation is especially important for overweight or obese children. As mentioned earlier, *perceived competence* is an important determinant of participation in physical activity and, also according to Albert Bandura, *self-efficacy* is an important determinant of how likely behavior is to change in general. Finding the right physical activity for your child takes time and patience:

Encourage your child, with your support, to try as many different physical activities as possible to find one that is sustainable.

A few years back, a financial services company offering retirement plans broadcast a humorous TV commercial featuring a high school basketball star who leads his team to a championship and is immediately offered a " seven-figure" contract to play for a professional team. His ecstatic father declares, "Son, we're going to be rich!" The basketball star responds, "But Dad, I don't want to play basketball. I want to dance." The son then breaks out into a musical dance routine. The father is forced to plan more carefully for his retirement. As lighthearted as that commercial was, it illustrates a couple of important points. First, too many parents often push their children into physical activities that *they* and not their children feel are rewarding. Start by asking your child what she is interested in. We've all heard stories of parents pursuing their own lost athletic opportunities vicariously through their children. Second, don't be afraid to "think outside the box" when it comes to helping your child find an enjoyable physical activity. There is nothing wrong with a boy who really wants to dance, fly a kite, or play lacrosse. The more different organized activities your child tries (within the limits of your resources, of course), the more likely it is that he will find one that he can sustain over a long period.

You should be present as your child tries new activities. Take an active role in the process. If you spot a soccer team practicing at a nearby field, for example, approach the coach and ask, "My daughter has never played soccer and is interested in trying it. Would it be possible for her to attend your next practice?" As she starts to participate, monitor her reaction to the activity carefully. Does she seem to enjoy it? Does it seem like she wants to go home? Are the other children making her feel welcome? After the activity, ask your child to tell you exactly how she feels. Ask her not only if she had a good time but also if she is looking forward to playing again. Gauge her perceived competence. Ask her if *she* felt she played well.

You may have to go through several different activities before finding at least one that is sustainable. Some physical activities may not be best for overweight or obese children to start with. Swimming, for example, may make an overweight or obese child self-conscious about his body. Activities that require a great deal of speed or stamina may discourage such a child from participating and may not be worth trying. Your child may enjoy a particular activity, but it may be too expensive or inaccessible to sustain. Common sense plays a big role in finding the right activity.

Family Meals and Good Feeding Habits

As I've mentioned, there are numerous benefits to regular family meals. Time constraints and difficult schedules sometimes make regular family meals impossible. Here are some tips to help you do the best you can.

Make family meals an experience your child values.

The family meal, even if it is hurried, should be an enjoyable experience. As noted, it is best to keep the TV off. Make a point of engaging your child in conversations about school, friends, or whatever else he feels like discussing. For older children, make attendance at family meals an important expectation: "No, you can't go over to your friend's house and grab something along the way because we're all about to have dinner together."

Take advantage of convenient but healthy options for family meals.

The "home meal replacement" market in the United States is growing very rapidly. As noted earlier, home meal replacements are generally healthier than the options available from inexpensive restaurants. Take advantage of them if you can. I realize that a "high-end" fresh home meal replacement for a family of four can cost $20 or more. The market, however, is becoming more competitive and this will, I hope, bring prices down. Almost all supermarkets offer less expensive frozen family dinners. These may not be quite as wholesome or tasty as the high-end meals, but they are far better than burgers and fries from a fast-food restaurant. (Even a frozen pizza without high-fat toppings such as pepperoni is a better option.) One major advantage of using frozen home meal replacements is that portion sizes are clearly marked. You should know precisely if your child is eating too much.

As the time available to prepare meals decreases, simple, fast-paced cooking (of the Jamie Oliver or Nigella Lawson variety) represents another healthy option. There are countless resources to help you in this regard. Among the best is the "minute meals" Web site: http://www.allfood.com/mmeal.cfm and the cookbook *Quick Meals for Healthy Kids and Busy Parents: Wholesome Family Recipes in 30 Minutes or Less from Three Leading Child Nutrition Experts.*[13]

Discontinue unhealthy feeding practices immediately.

The negative effects of unhealthy feeding practices should be clear to you by now. If your child complains, "I'm hungry," do not advise her to wait until dinner. Offer her a healthy snack such as a piece of fruit.

If your child tells you "I'm full," do not force her to eat any more than she wants to.

You may have noticed that apart from soft drinks, I've paid little attention so far to other types of so-called junk food such as packaged cakes, potato chips, ice cream, cookies, and other items. As opposed to soft drink consumption, no child can eat ice cream all day. I don't think it's wrong to indulge your child with such "junk food" once in a while. The key is to make junk food in your home seem like nothing special. Do not hide it in secret cupboards or keep it within sight but out of reach. Serve it on occasion as you would any other food. Do not restrict your child's intake. Allow her to have what she wants. This will prevent her from overeating the next time she comes across the same food. Older children may serve themselves or purchase their own junk food. This is a tougher situation since these children may have developed poor eating habits as a result of unhealthy feeding practices when they were younger. Try making healthy foods the "usual" snacks at home. Being a role model is also helpful. Avoid junk food yourself.

Keep Trying

You and your child will undoubtedly encounter setbacks. Reaching the goals in this chapter will require not only determination but also creativity. I've given you some tips on how to reach important goals. I encourage you and your child to develop your own strategies based on your experiences. Not being able to meet a goal in a reasonable period of time should not be perceived as a failure. It is only an opportunity to reflect, to rejuvenate, and, above all, to try again.

Chapter Ten

Advocacy for a Healthier "Built Environment"

I belong to several local and national organizations dedicated to fighting the childhood obesity epidemic. Some of these are research-oriented groups of professionals who meet periodically to discuss innovative approaches to the problem. Others have an educational mission to inform healthcare professionals and the general public about the seriousness of childhood obesity. The most unique are organizations that bring together physicians and other healthcare professionals, teachers, lawyers, community activists, and government officials in a common effort not to innovate or inform, but to try to convince powerful people and institutions to take specific action to create a healthier environment for America's children. In late 2004 I attended a childhood obesity "forum" with this theme in Pittsburgh. The first speaker was one of our local congressmen who was invited to share his perspective and also to listen to the many passionate voices in attendance. He started off by telling the group about how challenging it was to be a member of Congress, how hard he worked, and how little the general public understood about the workings of government. This irked just about everyone. He continued by telling us a story about how he had received a proposal to increase the number of bicycle paths in Pittsburgh to encourage physical activity. He said he initially thought it was a good idea but realized that there are only a limited number of federal funds available for infrastructure in our region.

"Did you know that Pittsburgh is the largest city in the United States without a beltway?"

He told us that a more senior conservative politician advised him that by voting for bicycle paths he would be jeopardizing the building of an Interstate beltway around metropolitan Pittsburgh. He concluded with some condescending remarks about how many people don't realize that "government cannot legislate good health." I was dumbfounded and angry. I wasn't alone. Several forum participants stood up immediately to challenge the congressman's remarks. Unfortunately, he left the room abruptly without facing a barrage of questions and criticism.

The congressman's remarks were ignorant. Beltways cost billions of dollars. Bicycle paths cost considerably less. The cities of Denver and Boulder, Colorado, are developing a bicycle path system for $8 million.[1] Actual need should determine the building of a beltway—not the fact that a city does not have one. Beltways are built to ease traffic congestion in and around cities and decrease the time required to get around a metropolitan area. Pittsburgh does have an extensive network of highways, though these do not form a circular beltway. Less time is lost by drivers in traffic delays in Greater Pittsburgh compared with any other metropolitan area its size in the United States.[2] Pittsburgh has among the lowest levels of traffic congestion in the country and congestion is increasing much more slowly than in almost any other city, owing in large part to the fact that the city's population is not increasing.[3] Pittsburgh is probably the best place right now *not* to build a beltway.

Why did I tell you about a congressman's lack of interest in funding bicycle paths? Recall that according to Albert Bandura behavior change depends both upon the "self" and the environment. As a parent, you have control over a large part of your child's environment. Your home, for example, can be made healthier by eliminating soft drinks. Obesity, however, is also a problem of the environment over which you do not have direct control and in which your child spends much of his time. This has been termed the "built environment" and refers to schools, parks, neighborhoods, and cities. Today the environment outside of your direct control has been called "obesigenic," because it can promote childhood obesity.

Unhealthy food is everywhere, including in schools. Physical education is being neglected in school curricula. The design of neighborhoods and cities discourages physical activity. If you try systematically to follow the recommendations in the previous chapter, you may come across one or more aspects of the built environment that prevents your child from achieving or maintaining a healthy weight. Your neighborhood, for example, may have few sidewalks, which may make a daily walk unsafe. While you can do an enormous amount to help your child, you cannot by yourself change the built environment. You need the support of those in positions who can. They are mostly school board members and elected officials at all levels of government. The congressman I told you about isn't unique. He illustrates the common lack of understanding of what contributes to obesity, of what the costs of childhood obesity are, and what constitutes a community's most pressing needs. This chapter is devoted to helping you become an agent of change to promote healthier communities by enlightening those with the power to take action.

WHY BECOME AN ADVOCATE?

The verb "advocate" is derived from the Latin word *advocare*, which means "to call to one's aid." An advocate's mission, therefore, is to help others. Your built environment may or may not help your child achieve or maintain a healthy weight. Many Americans live in well-planned neighborhoods with plenty of parks, sidewalks, sports facilities, and schools that promote a healthy lifestyle. If you are not among those lucky Americans, advocacy will help you and your child and other families in your community improve your environment. Advocacy should develop from a sense of collective responsibility. This is a feeling not everyone shares to the same extent. I am Canadian and Canadians are renowned for their sense of collective responsibility. I live in a region of the United States with an equally strong sense of collective responsibility. I think the vast majority of Americans have at least some desire to do something for the greater good. I don't think anyone has recently expressed this feeling better than Senator Barack Obama, the articulate, multicultural, rising political star who gave the opening address at the 2004 Democratic National Convention:

> If there's a child on the south side of Chicago who can't read, that matters to me, even if it's not my child. If there's a senior citizen somewhere who can't pay for her prescription and has to choose between medicine and the rent, that makes my life poorer, even if it's not my grandmother. If there's an Arab American family being rounded up without benefit of an attorney or due process, that threatens my civil liberties. It's that fundamental belief—I am my brother's keeper, I am my sister's keeper—that makes this country work. It's what allows us to pursue our individual dreams, yet still come together as a single American family. "E pluribus unum." Out of many, one.[4]

If your child has access to a built environment that promotes a healthy lifestyle and your child's friend does not, I believe that should provoke a sense that the situation is unjust. It doesn't allow your child's friend to live the same quality of life and reach his potential. Your community is poorer as a result. By becoming an advocate for a healthier community environment, you are doing your part to help all your community's children.

What if you don't feel a strong sense of collective responsibility? There are plenty of Americans who are able to provide their own children with all they need to be healthy and happy and feel they have no need to be advocates for a better built environment. They may feel that if other families would only work as hard to provide for their children as they have, there would be no need for collective responsibility and the policies and changes to the built environment that go along with it. Fortunately, the benefits of advocacy for a healthier environment should also appeal to them. The lawsuits against tobacco companies began in Mississippi a decade ago, not because of an outpouring of sympathy for the failing health of smokers, but because states were being forced to pay huge medical bills for smoking-related illnesses.[5] As I told you in chapter 1, the economic costs of obesity are enormous. An obese, sedentary child is likely to grow up to become an obese adult and to suffer obesity-related diseases, which ultimately we all pay for.

A healthier built environment does cost some money. Politicians, like our local congressman, often instinctively reject any proposal to invest in something whose benefits to them seem tenuous and in things that seem "green" or "alternative." I certainly believe that public funds should be invested wisely. That idea seems to have been thrown out the window in recent years. A congressman may be happy to invest in a multibillion-dollar beltway but not in a multimillion-dollar bicycle path system. Today's Washington politicians are the biggest spenders in forty years.[6] Some government spending actually promotes obesity. Some government agencies were set up to be champions of small businesses. The US Small Business Administration (SBA) was set up to provide capital and financing to small business entrepreneurs. Loans are supposed to be made to innovative small businesses to allow them to establish themselves and hopefully expand and create jobs. This is not how things have really worked. According to the Heritage Foundation, a conservative "think tank," in 1996, $1 billion of loans were made to new franchisees, mostly of chain fast-food restaurants.[7] Eric Schlosser asserts in his book *Fast Food Nation* that such franchises have a very high failure rate and much of the money is not recovered.[8] The net effect is that the American taxpayer is subsidizing large fast-food corporations and therefore promoting obesity and raising obesity-related costs. This twisted system is all disguised as a way to embrace true capitalism and help struggling entrepreneurs.

You should be an advocate for a healthier built environment to help your child and your neighbors' children live as well as possible— and to save all of us money in the long term. Failing to invest in a healthier environment is shortsighted and makes no sense, given that America today is wasting money in ways the Founding Fathers could not have imagined.

IMPORTANCE OF THE BUILT ENVIRONMENT

I've already told you that soft drinks, fast food, television, physical inactivity, and family meals all play an important role in contributing to childhood obesity. These are all things over which you as a parent can exercise a significant amount of control. To convince you that becoming an advocate for a healthier built environment is worthwhile, you also need to understand how much the built environment really matters. A systematic review published in 2002 showed that the level of physical activity among adults is strongly related to the availability of facilities such as bicycle paths and parks. Lack of such facilities strongly predicted lack of physical activity.[9] Another review in 2000 of physical activity among children found that high levels of physical activity were strongly associated with access to recreational facilities and programs.[10] A 2003 study compared the frequency of walking trips by adults in "high walkable" neighborhoods to the frequency in "low walkable" neighborhoods.[11] High walkable neighborhoods were safe and had a high density of houses, few dead-end streets, and stores and services in close proximity to residential areas. Adults in high walkable neighborhoods walked twice as often as those in low walkable areas.

The lesson is very clear: People of all ages are more active in an environment that makes physical activity more attractive. The evidence I have described so far, however, simply reports associations, and we are back to the same "chicken or egg" question I've mentioned earlier. Does a high walkable neighborhood make people walk more, or do people with a tendency to walk move into high walkable neighborhoods? Is the famous saying from the movie *Field of Dreams*, "If you build it, they will come," true? Fortunately, in this case there is evidence that changing the built environment (without changing its people) does increase physical activity. In 1996 the city of London improved its lighting along footpaths. Depending upon the footpath, use increased between 24 and 101% depending upon their location.[12] Adding bike lanes has been shown to increase bicycle use.[13] Redesign of a neighborhood in Hannover, Germany, to better accommodate both people and cars led to far more children playing actively on the street.[14]

Apart from facilities available for physical activity and walkable neighborhoods, there are other aspects of the built environment that influence physical activity. Surveys have shown that parents are very concerned about the safety of their neighborhoods when deciding whether and where to allow their children to play outside.[15] The two major safety concerns are crime and traffic. Strangely, it has not been shown consistently that the safety of neighborhoods is related to levels of physical activity among children. There may be a simple explanation for this. Unsafe neighborhoods are more likely to be poor. Children in poor neighborhoods are more dependent upon walking to get around, even when it's not safe. In other words, though unsafe neighborhoods are perceived to be an important barrier to physical activity, children in unsafe neighborhoods may have elevated levels of activity as a result of poverty and lack of motorized transportation.

The built environment not only refers to facilities for physical activity and walkability but also to what is known as the *community food environment*. This refers to the type and range of supermarkets, corner grocery stores, and restaurants available in a community. Unlike the clear benefits of an environment that promotes physical activity, it is unclear whether a healthy community food environment promotes healthy eating. A 1995 study in a poor Latino community, for example, revealed that residents preferred whole milk to low-fat milk, despite the widespread availability of low-fat milk in community stores.[16] The impact of a healthy community food environment needs further study. It makes sense, however, that people eat what is available for sale in close proximity. Inner-city communities in the United States are especially challenged in this respect. Supermarkets are scarce in the inner city; fast-food restaurants are plentiful. Small convenience stores, many of which are located in gas stations, are common. They sell lots of high-fat snack foods and little if any fresh fruit or vegetables. Inner-city residents pay considerably more for the same foods than residents of the suburbs. Creating a healthier community food environment in America's inner cities remains a significant challenge.

GETTING STARTED

If you are convinced that advocacy for a healthier built environment is worthwhile, there are many different ways to get started. I strongly believe that grassroots, community advocacy is most valuable. The targets of advocacy need to be well chosen and the approach should be diplomatic rather than antagonistic. I do not favor, for example, protesting against fast-food restaurants by picketing outside. Many fast-food restaurants are now responding to concerns about their products in response to market demand for healthier food rather than because of organized protests or lawsuits. Similarly, you are more likely to successfully advocate for healthier food in your child's school by sharing your knowledge of the information in this book and elsewhere, accompanied by gentle persuasion. A rational way to get started is to ask yourself questions about your own community:[17] Does the design of the neighborhood encourage physical activity? Do community facilities for entertainment and recreation exist, are they affordable, and do they encourage healthful behaviors? Can children pursue sports and other active-leisure activities without excessive concerns about safety? Are there tempting-yet-healthful alternatives to staying-at-home sedentary pastimes such as watching television? Are sound food choices available in local stores and at reasonable prices? Does your child's school provide a healthy food environment? Is physical education a significant part of your child's school's curriculum?

Once you have identified your community's shortcomings, you can start with a single, specific goal. As you pursue your goal, you are almost certainly going to run across many like-minded parents who will add weight to your cause. There is no universally successful formula for advocacy. Important lessons can be learned, however, from a couple of very successful cases.

BANNING SOFT DRINKS IN SCHOOLS

When I started writing this book, the movement to ban soft drinks in schools was sweeping across America. There are so many people trying to ban soft drinks in schools that it is impossible to keep track of each individual effort. California became the first state to ban soft drinks in all elementary and junior high schools.[18] As mentioned in chapter 2, banning soft drinks in schools, though no substitute for good parenting to eliminate soft drink consumption, is generally a good idea. After all, if your child's home is free of soft drinks, why shouldn't your child's school be as well? It is unfortunate that many schools still sell soft drinks, sometimes even during official meal times, in violation of USDA regulations.

With nearly 700,000 elementary, junior high, and high school students, the Los Angeles Unified School District (LAUSD) is the nation's second largest. It is also home to one of the first, large-scale efforts to ban soft drinks in school.[19] This wasn't the result of a single parent concerned about the health of children asking the school board to rid the schools of soft drinks. Parents were, however, critical members of a coalition that included teachers and principals, school board members, public health officials, healthcare professionals, and well-organized public health advocacy groups. As in almost every other effort to ban soft drinks in schools, those opposed to a ban in Los Angeles feared losing revenue from "pouring rights contracts." Soft drink companies sponsor events and provide merchandise that may otherwise be unavailable to students.

The coalition that won the battle to ban soft drinks raised a couple of powerful arguments against those opposed to a ban. First, schools have an important responsibility to improve the lives and prospects of children. This includes not only classroom education but also encouragement of physical activity and other healthy behaviors. Among all the things a school can do to improve the well-being of children, banning soft drinks is quite possibly the easiest. Consider how difficult it is to raise test scores in reading or prevent violence. Getting rid of soft drinks is an effective way to prevent obesity and its complications. As noted, caffeine, a common ingredient in most soft drinks, can cause restlessness, headaches, nausea, and insomnia in children. Many teachers have observed improvements in the attention span and energy level of students in schools that have banned soft drinks, though hard evidence for this is still lacking.

A second important argument raised by those in favor of a ban in Los Angeles addresses the issue of lost revenue. The health of children and the economics of schools are two separate issues that should not be mixed, according to Marlene Carter, an LAUSD board member who coauthored the policy of banning soft drinks.[20] This is a very important principle. In an ideal situation, the need to ban soft drinks and improve the health of children shouldn't have to be balanced against the need to generate revenue for schools. No one would accept that it would be all right to sell cigarettes in schools to children as long as it generated revenue. Why should they accept the sale of soft drinks for the same reason?

Additional convincing arguments to counteract the fear of lost revenue have been suggested by a group in San Francisco called Parents Advocating School Accountability (PASASF).[21] Many fears about lost revenue are raised by the soft drink companies themselves. The experience of PASASF and the Aptos Middle School in San Francisco dispels some important myths. First, schools need not necessarily lose money by banning soft drinks. Aptos Middle School replaced soft drinks with healthier alternatives, including bottled water, 100% fruit juice, and milk. Coke and Pepsi are two of the largest sellers of bottled water in the United States, through their Aquafina and Dasani brands. Sales of healthy drinks have the potential to make profits both for the companies that make them and for schools. Many companies claim that children won't purchase healthy drinks. PASASF points out that thirsty students will purchase what's available. The price of drinks is the most important determinant of drink selection. A high school in Minnesota replaced all but one of its ten soft drink machines with bottled water. The last machine contained both soft drinks and bottled water. When bottled water was priced at $0.75 and soft drinks were priced at $1.25, bottled water outsold soft drinks.

Some school officials point out that soft drink companies not only provide revenue to schools but also donate sports equipment, scoreboards, and other important items. It is not the duty of soft drink companies to fill in a void left by an inadequate public financing system for schools. Communities and their residents have a responsibility to make sure that schools are adequately funded.

Some people argue that banning soft drinks from schools takes away children's "right to free choice." This is, of course, a preposterous argument. Children are not free to choose many things in a school environment. Many schools include physical education in their curricula. Children are usually not free to choose not to participate in physical education classes. Allowing children to choose soft drinks in the name of freedom makes no sense. The argument that banning soft drinks takes away freedom is also hypocritical since soft drink companies sign exclusive pouring rights contracts with schools. A school or school district that signs a deal with one company doesn't allow its students to choose another's products. How does that represent the freedom to choose?

A movement to ban soft drinks in your child's school may already be under way. If not, it is relatively easy for you to get one started.

Health advocacy is rarely a lonely endeavor. You can easily enlist the support of other parents. Many school board officials may also have concerns about soft drinks in schools. Public health advocacy groups and the healthcare community are also on your side. The American Academy of Pediatrics, for example, strongly supports severely restricting access to soft drinks now and recommends that pediatricians work toward eliminating soft drinks in schools completely.[22] There is no precise formula for success. A good way to start is to write a letter signed by a group of concerned parents that takes advantage of what you have learned in this book and the lessons learned from other successful movements to ban soft drinks. Your letter should be addressed to the person most responsible for determining the availability of soft drinks, whether it be your school principal, the chair of the school board, or the school district official responsible for health and nutrition. Here is a template you can follow:

Dear _____:

We are writing as a group of concerned parents of children at _____ School. As you know, many schools and school districts across the country have completely banned the sale of soft drinks. There is strong evidence that soft drinks promote obesity and its consequences, poor dentition and behavioral problems. Banning soft drinks is among the simplest things a school can do to improve the health of its children. Thirsty children will purchase and drink what is available in school. Soft drinks should be replaced by healthier alternatives including bottled water, 100% fruit juices, and low-fat milk. Children will choose these alternatives when they are available.

I am aware that soft drinks companies contribute significantly to the financial well-being of _____ School. I believe strongly, however, that the school finances should not be balanced against the health of children. If _____ School and _____ School District is dependent upon revenues from soft drinks companies to provide a quality educational environment, this points to a flaw in public financing that should be solved in some other way. There is also evidence that fears of lost revenue are not justified. Healthy products can generate revenue that replaces the losses from soft drinks sales. The soft drinks companies themselves manufacture many healthy refreshments.

We are asking you to consider completely banning all sales of soft drinks in _____ School immediately. This action would not only align the school with other schools across the country but is also compatible with what is recommended by the American Academy of Pediatrics.

We look forward to meeting with you within the next couple of weeks and discussing this further.

Sincerely,

[Names]

This letter simply describes one approach to one problem. Parents of children at Aptos Middle School in San Francisco used a similar approach to improving the food that is offered in the school cafeteria. The same set of rules applies to many types of community health advocacy in which you can play a major role: (1) identify a problem accurately and systematically; (2) make sure you can articulate clearly why it is a problem; (3) find out what others have done to tackle the same problem; (4) anticipate resistance to solving the problem and be prepared to counteract arguments in favor of the status quo; (5) address your concerns to the most responsible party with the support of people and organizations with a similar perspective; and (6) make a clear request to discuss the problem in person with the responsible party. This adds necessary pressure and keeps the issue in the limelight.

THE PHYSICAL ENVIRONMENT

Creating a healthier physical environment for children is a challenge because it has to do with how space is allocated in a community.

Imagine that a new strip mall is opening up along a busy street. The owners of the strip mall want to purchase an adjacent couple of acres from the municipality to build a parking lot. This would allow customers to access the stores more easily and boost business. The municipal land is also ideal for a playground for children, in a community where playgrounds are scarce. The strip mall owners, of course, have no interest in purchasing the land to build a playground. That responsibility falls upon the municipality. The municipality is faced with the choice of selling the land for a tidy sum, not having to worry about developing it, and being able to collect property taxes indefinitely, or keeping the land, purchasing and maintaining playground equipment, foregoing tax revenue, and making sure that children are kept safe from traffic on the busy street. Looking at the choices from a purely financial perspective, the best option is obvious.

As in the case of ridding schools of soft drinks, winning the battle for a healthier physical environment requires separating profit from health.

Walking is the most popular, simplest, and cheapest form of physical activity. Not only does walking provide exercise, but also people often walk to get somewhere or do something (a walk to the store to buy milk, for example). Unfortunately, many American communities are simply not very walkable.

European visitors to the United States are astonished by the extent to which the automobile dominates transportation and the everyday lives of Americans. There are more than 200 million cars in America. The American Automobile Association (AAA) has an incredible 47 million members. Entire communities have been built around the needs of the automobile. Suburban sprawl is a direct result of that need. In many cases, driving from place to place has become a necessity. The cores of many American cities are either empty or inhabited only by those too poor to buy a piece of the suburban dream. The infrastructure needed to support a car culture is enormous and expensive. Much of it is supported by the public purse. The Interstate Highway System, for example, cost more than $300 billion to build.[23] Automobiles are responsible for a significant amount of air pollution and associated respiratory illnesses in American cities.[24] The cost to health of a car culture has also been shown to have an impact upon obesity. Residents in suburbs, where the density of housing is low, are heavier than those living in areas where the density of housing is high (e.g., central New York City and Boston).[25]

Some aspects of the car culture border on the ridiculous. The "drive thru" concept has gone overboard. You can buy a fast-food meal or withdraw money from your bank without leaving the driver's seat. In Pittsburgh, you can "drive thru" a beer distributor, place an order, and the attendant will put a case of beer in your trunk. At least one service that discourages getting out of your car is disappearing. Most gas stations in the United States and Canada no longer have full-service attendants, actually requiring customers to get out and pump their own gas. On the downside from a physical activity standpoint, most stations allow automatic payment at the pump, meaning that there is no need to walk even to the cashier.

The dominance of the automobile and its impact upon the use of space and upon public health are well known. What is truly sad is the degree to which pedestrians and cyclists have been relegated to second-class status. This is just beginning to change. Progressive communities across America are pushing "smart growth"—strategies to enhance the quality of life through land use that promotes denser, more environmentally friendly, and more walkable communities. A good and relatively inexpensive beginning is to make sure that children have safe routes to walk to school. In most communities, motivated children and parents can find one or more suitable organized physical activities, such as a soccer or basketball league. Making sure that a community is walkable, on the other hand, requires advocacy.

Many communities have set an important precedent by establishing safe walking or cycling routes to school. This makes the job of advocacy in your own community easier. If in a huge city like Chicago, with all its diverse neighborhoods and the hazards of traffic and crime, the majority of public school children can walk to school, why can they not do so in your community? If a safe route can be established for children to walk or bike to school, this improves the walkability (or bikeability) and the general health of the community. An assessment is the correct way to start. Walking to school may not be an option in many communities. In addition to concerns about traffic or crime, distance is a significant barrier to children walking to school in many communities.[26] A distance of a mile or less is a reasonable walk for most children. More than that may be difficult. It is my hope that there will be a more walkable America in the not too distant future where schools will be located closer to where children actually live. Even if your child's school is too far to walk, advocating for safe walking routes in general is a good idea. Experts recommend asking yourself the following questions to assess walking routes:[27]

- Are sidewalks and pathways clear of obstacles, in good condition, and continuous along the routes?
- Are there crosswalks and pedestrian signals at busy streets and intersections?
- Are curb ramps present at intersection crosswalks? Are they ADA (Americans with Disabilities Act) compliant?
- Do drivers yield to pedestrians at driveways and crosswalks?
- Is secure and convenient bicycle parking available at school?
- Is there sufficient operating width for bicycles along the route?
- Are curb radii too large, thus encouraging fast vehicle cornering?
- Do drivers, pedestrians, and bicyclists behave appropriately?
- Do routes provide adequate visibility, especially for pedestrians shorter than five feet tall?
- Are there adequate and visible signing and pavement markings?
- Is there enough lighting?

If your community doesn't meet these standards, it is time to take action. Surprisingly, simple and inexpensive changes in a community can improve the walking environment. These include the following:[28]

- Free up walkways and sight lines by trimming back plants and trees.
- Make pavement markings and other signage much more visible.
- Connect sidewalks and other walkways to provide for continuous pathways.
- Encourage "walking school buses" where children walk in a group to school.
- Promote cycling through "bicycle boulevards" where traffic-calming measures are put in place along routes to school to slow vehicular travel and reduce conflict points between bicyclists and motorists.
- Create or widen bicycle lanes.
- Push out the boundary of designated school zones.
- Increase the reach of safety education.

These improvements cost much less than what municipalities spend for, say, road maintenance or waste management. Concerns that changes to the environment designed to encourage walking are too expensive are hard to justify. I would use the general approach to advocacy I outlined earlier. In addition to the support of other parents, the movement to establish safe walking routes is growing rapidly, and excellent information resources are available, including the Pedestrian and Bicycle Information Center (http://www.bicyclinginfo.org).[29]

SUCCESS BREEDS SUCCESS

Successfully reaching one or two specific goals through community advocacy is likely to inspire more efforts and more successes. If you can successfully advocate for safe walking routes to school, why not advocate for more green space where children can play? If you can get your school or school district to ban soft drinks, why not advocate for more mandatory physical education? A single successful effort can lead to the development of coalitions that can advocate for a wide range of improvements to build healthier communities. The cost of becoming a health advocate is small; the potential benefits are enormous. For the sake of your child, your family, and your community, I urge you to get started.

Chapter Eleven

A Glimpse of the Future

The term "futurism" was first used to describe an artistic movement that began in Italy in the early twentieth century. Futurism glorified twentieth-century life. Paintings, sculptures, and literature depicted machinery and the industrial age.[1] Today, the terms "futurism" and "futurist" are much less specific. Anyone with a vision of the future based upon science, historical precedent, conjecture, prophecy, or any combination of these has called himself a futurist. In trying my hand as a futurist, I would like to share some thoughts here about the future care of overweight and obese children based upon recent and forthcoming developments and my own convictions about what is likely to succeed and how society will respond to this worsening problem. The original futurism showed us the glory of machines. It is unfortunate that those machines have contributed to today's childhood obesity epidemic.

There are two important things I believe about the future that are different from some other experts in the field of obesity. First, as mentioned earlier, I am optimistic that the problem of childhood obesity will eventually be brought under control. In contrast to the original futurism, I am hopeful that a future where children rely less on machines to get around and eat less food that is prepared by machines is on its way. I do not believe that today's generation of children will be the first not to outlive its parents.

In an article in *Time* magazine titled "Visions of the 21st Century: Will We Keep Getting Fatter?" journalist Michael Lemonick writes, "We'll keep getting fatter and fatter, with no real prospect of reversing the trend. Unless medical science provides a quick fix, that is."[2] Not only do I not share Mr. Lemonick's pessimism, but I also do not believe that a "quick fix" or "magic bullet" will be the ultimate solution to the problem. I've emphasized throughout this book that there is currently no magic bullet for the problem of obesity. In the foreseeable future, I do not predict the widespread availability of a simple, effortless, safe remedy for children. Even if such a remedy ever does become available, it will be many more years before the problem of obesity is solved. Simple "magic bullet" solutions have eliminated some public health problems over a long period of time. The smallpox vaccine, for example, successfully eradicated smallpox worldwide by the 1970s. Compared to obesity, smallpox was a relatively simple problem. Edward Jenner first developed a crude smallpox vaccine in the late 1700s. Thus it took nearly two hundred years for humankind to solve a relatively simple public health problem.

I believe that childhood obesity will eventually be brought under control primarily through changes in the built environment (neighborhoods, schools, foods available in convenience stores, etc.). Such changes will both prevent and treat childhood obesity. A number of new medications for the treatment of obesity will become available in the coming years. I believe they will be used to treat a relatively small proportion of obese children. I also believe that refinements in behavioral and surgical approaches will allow another small proportion of obese children to achieve a healthy weight.

A BUILT PHYSICAL ENVIRONMENT FOR THE
NEW MILLENNIUM: SPRAWL AND SMART GROWTH

I went to a conference in Orlando, Florida, a couple of years ago and stayed at a hotel a half mile away from the conference site. The first morning of the conference I asked a hotel clerk for directions to the conference center. She said she would be happy to call for a taxi. "Can't I just walk there?" I asked.

"Hmm. I don't think so. I've never heard of anyone doing it."

Undaunted and on such a beautiful day, I decided to give it a try. I could see the conference center from the hotel parking lot across several broad avenues and huge concrete barriers lined with palm trees. There were no sidewalks or crosswalks anywhere. Cars zipped by at fifty or sixty miles an hour. The hotel clerk was right: it wasn't possible to walk. "You can't walk there from here" applies to many communities all across America. It is largely the result of urban sprawl—the rapid, uncontrolled, poorly planned spread of homes and businesses beyond the original boundaries of cities.

Sprawl has many causes. According to the 1996 documentary *Taken for a Ride*,[3] the big three American automobile manufacturers and others lobbied aggressively for building highways that contributed to sprawl. It became possible for people to live far from where they worked. When given a choice between a nice piece of land in the suburbs or a crowded plot in the city, many chose the former. The well-documented phenomenon of "white flight" is also responsible for sprawl. As African Americans migrated to cities across America in large numbers in the thirties, forties, and fifties, many white families elected to segregate themselves by building what was then considered a suburban utopia.

Whatever its root causes, many Americans have come to realize that sprawl is not a good thing. Low-density development of homes and businesses far from city centers not only encourages obesity through reliance on the automobile but also has a more general, negative impact on quality of life. Atlanta is America's most sprawling city.

Atlantans endure the longest commute times in the country. Sitting in a car on a clogged highway surrounded by hot, smog-filled air is not the best way to spend one's time. Furthermore, sprawling low-density development is actually more expensive for municipalities and states to maintain. In Maine, for example, public school enrollment fell by twenty thousand between 1970 and 1995. Because of sprawl, however, the state spent $338 million to build new schools.[4] A smaller number of children was spread thinner. The "Smart Growth" movement is the result of frustration with sprawl.

"Smart growth" is the efficient use of land to create or revitalize communities to include transportation choices, open spaces, recreational and educational opportunities, a range of housing alternatives, and commercial services and other businesses in a single area. In an ideal "smart growth" neighborhood, it would be possible to walk to school, walk to a friend's house, walk to a supermarket, walk to a barber, and walk to a baseball diamond or a tennis court. The "smartest" city in America is Portland, Oregon. Portland has an "urban growth boundary" to prevent sprawl. Development beyond the boundary is not permitted. This forces developers to come up with innovative, higher-density developments that are more likely to meet the smart growth ideal. Portland also has excellent public transportation and 221 miles of bicycle paths that allow cyclists to commute downtown safely.[5]

Unfortunately, most American cities are far less progressive and are more likely to resemble Atlanta than Portland. I believe, however, that frustration with sprawl will reach a breaking point and that more and more Americans will embrace smart growth. Citizens, architects, urban planners, developers, environmentalists, public health professionals, and governments, at all levels, are finally coming together to determine how best to develop vibrant, healthy communities all across the country. It may take fifty years or more for the phenomenon of sprawl to finally end, but the process is beginning. As a welcome sign, the populations of the downtowns of almost all of America's largest cities are expected to rise dramatically by 2010.[6] Middle-class and upper-middle-class Americans are choosing high-density, downtown living as an alternative to life in the suburbs. Gradually, the new downtown dwellers are demanding all the amenities of the suburbs but located in a compact area. It is somewhat ironic that this type of new, progressive smart growth based on revitalization of city centers is actually recreating what American cities were like many years ago. Obesity was much less of a problem in the smarter cities of the past than it is today. Smart growth of the future will help keep kids slimmer.

THE COMING COMMUNITY FOOD ENVIRONMENT

I do not predict the demise of fast-food restaurants or the unavailability of regular soft drinks in the near future. I believe that the large companies that control much of the community food environment will continue to respond to public pressure, however, by offering healthier alternatives. Many schools are leading the way by replacing soft drinks and other "competitive" foods with bottled water and healthy snacks. A healthy community food environment is already becoming "fashionable" among some segments of the population. Whole Foods, for example, caters to sophisticated, urban professionals. Being fat has never been fashionable, and as more Americans come to understand the role of fast food and other junk food in the childhood obesity epidemic, more Americans will opt for healthier food in their communities.

I also believe that many Americans will view a healthy community food environment as socially just. The inner-city neighborhood in which my practice is located is full of fast-food restaurants. Poor African Americans are among their best customers. The poor, especially those from certain minority groups, suffer disproportionately from obesity. I believe that Americans from poor communities in rural and urban America should and will demand a healthier and affordable community food environment. The Whole Foods Market in Pittsburgh is located in an inner-city neighborhood, but few of its customers actually live there. Why should only the well-to-do eat well as fast-food companies make fat profits while making the poor fat? Across the country the inner-city poor have lobbied, often successfully, for better housing, jobs, public transportation, and better schools. I believe they will also lobby for a healthier community food environment. The quality of available food has an enormous impact upon the health of children and families. I predict that a healthy community food environment will be available to everyone within ten to fifteen years.

Health policy specialists and nutrition advocates have proposed several ideas to encourage consumption of healthier food. The idea of a tax on junk food has been around for several years. A special tax would be imposed upon unhealthy foods such as potato chips. The money collected would be used for health promotion campaigns or to subsidize healthy foods such as fruits and vegetables. Americans have a natural aversion to new taxes. Whether such a tax would have its intended effect is uncertain. Michael Jacobsen (author of the "Liquid Candy" report) and Kelly Brownell reviewed the idea in a paper published in 2000.[7] Many states and some municipalities do currently tax soft drinks and unhealthy snacks. Few jurisdictions, however, use the money for health promotion. None use the money to subsidize healthy food. Tennessee, for example, uses some of its soft drink tax revenue to clean up highways, which is a worthwhile aim but does not address the problem of obesity.

Even small taxes on soft drinks and other junk foods can generate a significant amount of money. A national one cent per 12-oz. serving of soft drink tax would generate an estimated $1.5 billion annually. This is not enough money to bring down the price of fresh fruits and vegetables through subsidies, but it is enough to fund educational campaigns that encourage healthy eating. A community-based seven-week educational campaign in Clarksburg, West Virginia, was successful in boosting the local market share of low-fat milk, as opposed to higher-fat milk, from 18 to 41%.[8] The campaign cost just twenty-two cents per each resident.

Whether a hefty tax on unhealthy foods is a good idea that would curb childhood obesity is unclear. Many companies are obviously opposed to it. One of the major questions is exactly which foods would be taxed and which would be exempt. Still, I do not predict widespread taxes on junk food anytime soon. I believe, however, that the companies that make unhealthy foods may find another idea more appealing.

The Coca-Cola and Pepsi companies began introducing "low-carb" versions of their products a couple of years ago. These are just like regular colas but have half the high-fructose corn syrup. The new products are popular because they don't taste like diet soft drinks and are lower in calories than regular soft drinks. The soft drink companies are simply responding to market demand for "low-carb" products, just as McDonald's is now profitably offering healthier alternatives on its menu. Companies that do introduce healthier items, however, do take a significant financial risk.

Rather than taxing unhealthy foods, how about a tax break for the development of healthy versions of what are now unhealthy foods? Fast-food restaurants, for example, take a major risk when they develop and market new items. In 1991 McDonald's promoted ten new menu items. Only two remain on the menu today.[9] Some healthier products, such as the low-fat "McLean Deluxe" burger, sold poorly. Snack-food companies have also suffered the same way. Sales of Fat Free Pringles and Wow potato chips (that use a type of fat that is not absorbed) have been poor.[10] Developing healthy products that customers will actually find tasty and that generate profits is a big challenge for companies that have relied on steady sales of unhealthy foods for years. To encourage the development of such products, I thus propose that companies should be permitted to deduct a portion of the development and marketing cost. This would make introducing healthy products less risky. I also believe that with increasing consciousness of the problem of obesity, especially obesity among children, some healthy products would sell well. Imagine a new Big Mac made with leaner meat and a thinner, whole-grain bun and topped with fresh vegetables without any "special sauce." It would have a third or more fewer calories than its old counterpart. These days I think many people would buy it.

OBESITY DRUGS

Much media attention about obesity is devoted to news about new drugs that promote weight loss. The drug treatment of obesity does not have a good track record. There are two principal problems that have come up consistently for decades. First, the effectiveness of some widely marketed obesity drugs is questionable. Second, most drugs developed to date have serious side effects.[11] Thyroid hormone was the first drug used to treat obesity. Excessive thyroid hormone given alone is associated with heart rhythm disturbances and even sudden death. In the 1940s through the 1960s, amphetamines were prescribed for obesity, often in combination with thyroid hormone. The combination was associated with addiction, high blood pressure, and sudden death.[12] The most recent obesity drug fiasco is the combination of fenfluramine-phentermine, commonly known as "fen-phen." This drug acted on the brain to reduce appetite. Fen-phen was introduced in 1992. In 1996 the first reports of a rare condition called *primary pulmonary hypertension* among some patients on fen-phen began to surface. Primary pulmonary hypertension is incurable and normally kills only 125 to 150 Americans a year. It is characterized by increases in blood pressure in the arteries of the lungs that causes the heart to fail and eventually causes death.[13] Fen-phen was also associated with serious abnormalities of the heart valves. The drug was pulled off the market in September 1997.[14] Even widely available over-the-counter drugs for weight loss have been associated with serious problems. Phenylpropanoloamine (found in Accutrim™ and Dexatrim™) was pulled off the market in 2000 because it significantly elevates the risk of stroke.[15]

Drugs for the treatment of obesity fall into three categories: drugs that decrease appetite through their action on the brain; drugs that increase metabolism so that more energy is burned; and drugs that act on the intestines to decrease absorption of energy. At the present time only two drugs, sibutramine (Meridia™) and orlistat (Xenical™), are approved for the long-term treatment of obesity. Neither is approved for treatment in children.

Sibutramine acts on the brain to decrease appetite through its action on norepinephrine and serotonin, two important components of the brain's chemistry. A systematic review of the effectiveness of sibutramine published in 2004[16] reveals average weight losses of roughly six pounds after three months of use and ten pounds after one year of use. Sibutramine appears to be safe although it causes slight increases in blood pressure in some patients.[17] I have prescribed it to a small number of adult patients who have obesity-related diseases, since even modest weight loss can improve some conditions. For the majority of obese patients, however, taking a drug for an entire year to lose about ten pounds just isn't going to make a lot of difference.

Orlistat acts on the intestines to block the breakdown of fat. Since the fat is not broken down, the body cannot absorb it. The drug itself is not absorbed by the bloodstream. For this reason it is thought to be safer than many other drugs. Taking orlistat is like coating the intestines with a special substance that prevents only fat from being absorbed into the body. Since fat contains lots of calories, orlistat promotes weight loss. In studies comparing orlistat to placebo, subjects taking the drug lost 5.9 to 10% of their original weight compared to 4.6 to 6.4% among patients taking placebo over one to two years.[18] For a person weighing 200 lbs., this translates to a weight loss with orlistat of 12 to 20 lbs. This is a modest amount that can be important for people with obesity-related diseases. Unfortunately, orlistat is frequently associated with loose, oily bowel movements that can be bothersome to some.[19] Since orlistat blocks the absorption of fat, people already eating a low-fat diet are unlikely to benefit that much.[20]

Because it is relatively safe and produces respectable weight losses over time, orlistat is the only drug that is receiving serious consideration as a treatment in children at this time. A large National Institutes of Health (NIH) study is now under way to determine the effectiveness of orlistat in producing weight loss in obese African American and Caucasian children ages 12 to 17 who have at least one obesity-related illness such as high blood pressure, type 2 diabetes, high cholesterol, or sleep-related breathing problems. The Food and Drug Administration requires three levels of testing prior to approval of any drug. In *Phase I* clinical trials, a drug is evaluated for the first time to assess its safety and to identify side effects in a small number of patients. In *Phase II* clinical trials, the drug is administered to a larger number of patients to assess both its effectiveness and safety. In *Phase III* trials, the drug is given to a very large number of people (often one thousand to three thousand) to confirm its effectiveness, to monitor side effects, and most important, when possible, to compare it to other treatments. A phase I trial of orlistat has been completed in adolescents and the drug has proven to be safe and tolerable in the short term.[21]

The diabetes drug metformin has been used in Europe for nearly thirty years and was approved for use in the United States in 1995. In addition to reducing blood sugar levels, metformin has been shown in some studies to promote weight loss. Other studies have shown little or no weight loss or an inconsistent effect across different patients. A large study to evaluate the effectiveness of metformin in promoting weight loss in obese adolescents without diabetes is now under way.[22] At the present time, metformin is approved only as a diabetes drug.

The greatest promise for effective drugs for the treatment of obesity comes from improved understanding of the complex hormones that control body weight through their effect on the nervous system. This has been a field of intense research for some time. Different hormones either increase or decrease appetite by acting on different cells in the brain. The processes involved are very complicated.[23] A few key conclusions drawn from years of research will suffice for our purposes here. Four hormones largely regulate appetite. Fat tissue produces *leptin*. Leptin acts on the brain to stimulate nerve cells that decrease appetite. The pancreas produces *insulin*, which has a similar effect on the brain. The intestines produce *cholecystokinin*, which also decreases appetite but by stimulating nerve fibers in the stomach as well as by acting in the brain. Finally, the hormone *ghrelin* is produced by the stomach and acts in the brain to increase appetite. In summary, leptin, insulin, and cholecystokinin decrease appetite and promote weight loss; ghrelin increases appetite and promotes weight gain. Much about insulin has been known for a long time. You will hear a great deal more about leptin, cholecystokinin, and ghrelin, however, in the coming years.

Researchers are trying to develop drugs that influence the effects of these hormones and therefore promote weight loss. A drug that boosts the effect of cholecystokinin, for example, can be expected to decrease appetite and weight. Though improved understanding of the hormones that regulate body weight is valuable, results of studies based on this understanding have not always yielded positive results. Giving people synthetically produced leptin might seem like an effective cure for obesity. Results of studies using leptin as a treatment, unfortunately, have been generally disappointing, although some people appear to respond to the hormone with significant weight loss.[24]

The next drug likely to be approved for the treatment of obesity is *rimonabant*. It blocks cannabinoid receptors in the brain (the same receptors that respond to marijuana) and decreases appetite. Precisely how it works is unclear, but an effect on the hormone ghrelin is suspected.[25] A recent large phase III trial showed that rimonabant causes an average weight loss of roughly twenty pounds over two years among adult patients with obesity-related diseases.[26] The drug may also help people quit smoking. Rimonabant is being hailed by some as a miracle cure for obesity that will generate huge profits for its manufacturer. It has received an enormous amount of attention in the general media. *BusinessWeek*, for example, published a story in 2004 titled "Has Obesity Met Its Match?"[27] The drug may be available for sale this year.

IMPORTANT LESSONS ABOUT OBESITY DRUGS

In general, I am deeply skeptical about the development of safe, effective drugs for the treatment of obesity *in children*. The fen-phen story is only the latest of a long series of disasters. There are several reasons for the poor track record of obesity drugs. Millions of people are desperate to lose weight, and the pharmaceutical industry has the potential to reap huge profits from the sale of an effective treatment for obesity. I believe that these factors create a sense of urgency that can lead to errors at many levels. Pharmaceutical companies aggressively promote current and future weight-loss drugs that generate excitement and hope. The FDA is coming under increasing criticism for responding to pressure to speed up the approval of drugs while failing to adequately monitor safety. Patients hear about miracle cures for obesity on the way and demand them from drug companies and physicians, which generates more pressure.

The hype over obesity drugs often overshadows three important questions about any weight-loss drug. First, how effective is it? To date, most drugs have produced modest amounts of weight loss. A drug will not make a very obese person thin. This brings up the second important question. Who can benefit most from the drug? The answer is usually people who have obesity-related diseases in whom even a modest amount of weight loss can bring these diseases under better control. Finally, what are the risks of taking the drug? The risks must always be weighed against the benefits. A modest amount of weight loss may not be worth the risk of potential heart problems. I believe that these questions will remain unanswered about future obesity drugs for many years to come. Obese adults with obesity-related diseases will be the targets of almost all future therapies. The makers of rimonabant, for example, are seeking approval for its use only in obese adults who have obesity-related diseases such as diabetes. The lessons for drug treatment in children are clear. The number of obesity drugs approved for use in children is likely to remain small for many years. Such drugs will be used to treat a very small number of children with significant obesity-related diseases such as diabetes who can benefit from modest amounts of weight loss. Concerns about safety may emerge even after a drug is approved. For the majority of obese children, drugs are not and will not be the answer any time in the foreseeable future.

SURGICAL TREATMENT OF OBESITY

For some very obese patients, surgery is the answer. The surgical treatment of obesity is known as *bariatric surgery*. About 16,000 bariatric surgeries were performed in the United States in 1992; 103,000 were performed in 2003.[28] The two most common types of surgery performed today are the *gastric bypass* and *gastric banding*. The gastric bypass involves creating a small pouch out of the existing stomach through which food passes. The pouch is then connected to the intestines. The net effect is to create a new smaller stomach that holds less food. The original stomach is therefore "bypassed." The gastric band uses a similar principle. A band is wrapped around the outside of the stomach to reduce its size. The band can be adjusted to different levels of tightness. Both procedures make it difficult to eat large amounts and therefore promote weight loss. Both procedures are now largely performed *laparoscopically*, meaning through the use of a camera and small incisions through which long instruments are inserted. Gastric bypass was originally mostly performed through large incisions that exposed much of the abdominal cavity. Patients recover quicker from laparoscopic surgery. The adjustable gastric band is thought to be safer than gastric bypass because it doesn't involve actually cutting part of the stomach. The adjustable band also allows the size of the stomach to be adjusted to allow for gradual rather than rapid weight loss.

Bariatric surgery is associated with significant and sometimes dramatic weight loss in very obese patients. There are, however, major risks. Serious complications, including death, are not uncommon.[29]

The surgery is best performed by experienced surgeons in centers where specialized expertise in nutrition and psychology are available. Only a small number of children, all of them adolescents, have undergone bariatric surgery in the United States. Experts in the field have raised concerns about the impact of bariatric surgery on growth and development, future fertility, and the development of eating disorders.[30] For these reasons, strict guidelines have been adopted to determine which adolescents should have surgery. Adolescents must meet *all* of the following criteria:[31]

- Have tried six or more months of weight management through other methods and have not succeeded in losing weight.
- Have gone through or have nearly gone through all of puberty.
- Have a BMI of 40 or more and obesity-related diseases or a BMI of 50 or more without obesity-related diseases.
- Able to undergo medical and psychological evaluations prior to and after surgery, and to follow nutritional guidelines after surgery.
- Able to make informed decisions about treatment and have a supportive family environment.

I am impressed that such a cautious approach to bariatric surgery in adolescents is being promoted. I believe that a very small number of adolescents who meet the criteria will continue to benefit immensely from surgery. I don't believe that surgery will become a common treatment for the majority of obese children anytime in the near future.

THE FUTURE OF BEHAVIORAL TREATMENTS

I believe that changing eating and physical activity behaviors based on the principles I've described in chapter 8 will remain the most popular approaches to childhood obesity for a long time. I am also optimistic that a few approaches that one can only describe as "unorthodox" will consistently prove effective. I told you, for example, that the Cochrane Collaboration has found that "relaxation" is an effective therapy for obesity. The evidence, however, comes from just one study in Germany in which children were enrolled in a standard behavioral program or a program that included muscle relaxation techniques.[32]

Progressive muscle relaxation is among the most common muscle relaxation techniques. It involves voluntarily tensing and relaxing muscles in sequence from the head to the feet. A common way to start is to raise the eyebrows as high as possible and then to relax them after "tension builds." The technique is promoted for the treatment of stress, insomnia, and a host of other disorders as well as for obesity. The German investigators found, by accident, that muscle relaxation was more effective as a treatment for obesity than expected. Their results have not been confirmed by others. It is unfortunate that such simple and safe approaches to weight loss do not receive the huge media attention of emerging obesity drugs, nor the funding necessary to carry out more studies to prove their effectiveness.

Chapter Twelve

Stories of Three Children

We've covered a great deal of ground, and I hope you are eager to put it to good use. This chapter will give you some practice before you use what you've learned to help your own child. I've been involved in medical education for several years. I've developed an interest in developing innovative ways for medical students, medical residents, and practicing physicians to learn better. Case studies have been used as a successful learning method in many different professional disciplines, including law, business, and medicine. In 1997 I developed a new format for medical case studies that begins with a brief summary of a patient's life story. The story is followed by detailed medical information and questions about how to care for the patient for the reader to consider, either alone or as part of a discussion group. I used this format in my textbook for medical students, *Primary Care Management: Cases and Discussions*.[1] Learning through cases has some distinct advantages over other ways to learn. The renowned psychologist Carl Rogers wrote in 1961 that "the only learning that significantly influences behavior is self-discovered, self-appropriated learning."[2] Case studies fit this standard. A well-written case study encourages a reader to discover relevant facts and apply important principles to his own learning needs.

Based on the format I developed, I've included brief stories of three children. I begin each story with a description of each child that includes some essential details for you to consider. I follow this with a couple of questions I'd like you to consider carefully before moving on. The final part of each story tells you what each child and his or her family did to help each child on his or her way to becoming fit, trim, and happy. These stories are composites of real patients. I've tried to roll my experience in caring for many overweight and obese children into three representative children. Each story doesn't include all the lessons from chapter 9. Collectively, however, I've tried to illustrate many important lessons. Bear in mind that it isn't possible for a family to do everything for their child all at once. Some of you may find that your child has a lot in common with the children I describe.

EMILY'S STORY

High school has been unkind to Emily. She and her family moved to Glen Ridge just six months ago. She began tenth grade not knowing a soul in a stable community where most of her classmates had known each other since elementary school. Emily has always been painfully shy. Her new surroundings have made her feel even more withdrawn and lonelier than usual. She has no close friends, though she walks to school with her twelve-year-old brother, Danny, and Danny's friend Jay.

Emily is not involved in sports, music, or any clubs either in or outside of school. Her parents have tried hard, without much success, to encourage her to participate in some extracurricular activity. The family has followed the same hapless type of effort for years. Recently, for example, when Emily's little brother started taking judo lessons, Emily's mother asked the instructor if there was a class for her fifteen-year-old daughter too. She persuaded Emily to sign up. After one introductory lesson, Emily came home and told her mother, "Mom, that just isn't for me. I'm not going anymore."

Emily and her family have a very predictable daily routine. Emily gets off the school bus at 4 PM. Her younger brother returns around the same time. She is supposed to "keep an eye on him" until her parents get home, but she usually heads straight to her room. Emily's father, Peter, is an accountant and leaves for work early in the morning and returns home at six. Emily's mother, Barbara, is a nurse at an assisted-living facility. She always works in the daytime and returns home around five. In her bedroom, Emily boots up her computer and starts "chatting" online. This is how she spends almost all her free time. Emily has plenty of friends in the "cyberworld" from all over the globe. She bears her soul to a fifteen-year-old boy in England, who promises to marry her some day. A thirteen-year-old girl from Argentina helps her with her Spanish homework. In her cyberworld Emily lives vicariously as a popular, bold, beautiful teenager. In the chat rooms she is the center of attention. Very little distracts Emily from her computer. She usually brings a bowl of chips, grated cheddar cheese, some salsa, and a bottle of soda with her upstairs. Emily's parents rarely cook. They bring home takeout (especially Chinese) at least three days a week. Barbara's pleas of "Emily, dinner's ready" are either met with silence or "Mom, I'm doing homework. I'll eat later." This part about homework is seldom true. Emily's grades reflect a lack of attention to homework and schoolwork in general.

Emily does indeed eat later—often much later. Stuffed with chips and cheese, she doesn't usually get hungry again until about nine o'clock. That's when she scrounges through the kitchen, preparing a plate that includes leftovers, chips, cookies, and fruit cocktail. She eats this peculiar mélange while chatting online, often late into the night. She rarely gets to bed before midnight.

Emily stands 5'7" and weighs about 210 lbs. She has gained nearly thirty pounds since moving to Glen Ridge. At a recent checkup, her family doctor expressed concern about her blood pressure, which was slightly elevated above normal.

Questions for You to Consider

What do you think is contributing most to Emily's weight problem?

What specific changes do you believe that Emily and her family could make to help her achieve a healthy weight?

ON HER WAY TO A HEALTHIER WEIGHT

What contributed to Emily's obesity should be fairly obvious. She is not physically active at all. Her diet consisted largely of junk food including soft drinks. It wouldn't be surprising if she purchased junk food at school for lunch. She spent an enormous amount of time in front of her computer including before bedtime. She had poor sleep habits. The family meal environment was not compatible with a healthy weight. Emily and her family thus had a great deal of work to do.

Emily's personality and loneliness were probably both among the causes and the consequences of her weight problem. She was socially very isolated. She found solace on the Internet. Her time on the computer and her eating habits contributed to her obesity, and this in turn made her feel even more like she didn't belong among children in her neighborhood. She retreated further from classmates and her family into the "cyberworld."

Peter and Barbara decided finally to help Emily break free of the vicious circle of social isolation, computer addiction, and poor eating habits. They knew that they couldn't solve all Emily's problems at once. They began by setting a few broad, behavioral goals: Emily was to be more physically active; she was to reduce her time on the computer; she was to eliminate consumption of regular soft drinks. Peter and Barbara next asked Emily to record exactly how much time she spent on her computer each day as honestly and accurately as possible for a week. She was also expected to record how much soda she normally drinks. The results were surprising, even to Emily. Emily was online an average of seven hours per day. She drank roughly one liter of soda a day, the equivalent of roughly 450 calories.

Barbara next took the initiative to establish a family-walking program. Barbara, Emily, and Danny now walk together around their neighborhood for one mile every evening no matter what the weather. Danny is not overweight, but Barbara insisted that he join the walks so that Emily doesn't feel "singled out." (Sometimes Danny chooses to ride his bike along instead of walking.) Barbara and Emily have been enjoying the walks immensely. Barbara's normally reticent daughter has gradually opened up about a number of things that are important to her.

Peter has been especially concerned about Emily's lack of involvement in extracurricular activities. One evening, with the all kindness of a loving father, he asked, "Sweetheart, I know what Danny likes to do, but you never tell me what you like. Please let me know."

"Dad, I want to take up painting," Emily responded.

"Okay. That's good. Let's make it happen. Do you like any sports? I know you've tried soccer, basketball, tennis, and judo. Do you think you'd like something else?"

"Some of those sports make you run too much. I can't keep up. Nobody makes fun of me. I mean the other girls are really nice, but I feel like I'm letting everyone down. I think judo is just plain scary. I didn't like it at all."

Peter pressed her. "Okay. We'll stay away from those sports. There are lots of others you know."

"I know, Dad. Most sports make you wear shorts. My legs are huge. I feel really uncomfortable. There's a girl in my algebra class who goes bowling with her mother. She told me once I could come along. It sounds like fun."

"Bowling, huh? Well, that wouldn't have been my first choice, but if that's what you like, I think you should definitely go."

Emily, her new friend Jennifer, and Jennifer's mother now go bowling about twice per week. Emily has a great time. It may not be the most physically demanding of sports, but Peter and Barbara are happy that their daughter has found something she's interested in that at least keeps her moving. Respecting her wishes, Peter enrolled Emily in a painting class through a city recreational program. There, Emily has gradually opened up to other children and is starting to make some meaningful friendships.

Barbara has taken the initiative to reduce the amount of junk food at home. The soda has been replaced with skim milk. Chips and cookies have been replaced with apples. Danny complained about this for a few weeks but now reaches for fresh fruit whenever he wants a snack.

With her new activities, Emily's computer time has gone down to roughly 2–3 hours a day. The soda she drank is high in caffeine. Eliminating it has helped Emily sleep better. The family is still struggling to create a healthier family meal environment.

Slowly and steadily, Emily has lost weight. Six months after Peter and Barbara made a commitment to help her achieve a healthy weight, Emily weighs 184 lbs. (a loss of 26 lbs.). Her blood pressure is normal. Her confidence has improved, and she has expressed an interest in taking up dancing.

DARRYL'S STORY

Anyone who meets Darryl would describe him as quite a character. Known to his friends at school as a prankster, Darryl has managed to stay out of trouble by winning over his teachers and classmates with his charm. On his most recent report card, Darryl's homeroom teacher wrote, "Darryl is an average student. I think he could do better if he would take his schoolwork more seriously and stopped joking around as much. That having been said, I sure will miss Darryl next year!"

Darryl is an eleven-year-old African American boy who lives with his mother, Glenda, and nine-year-old sister, Taja, in an apartment in the Hamlin Park area of Buffalo, New York. Darryl's parents divorced when he was seven. Glenda works as a receptionist for an insurance company. Early in the school year she received a note from a school nurse who expressed her concern about Darryl's weight. The nurse included a pamphlet about healthy eating habits. Darryl is 4'10" tall and weighs 135 lbs. His BMI is 28.3 kg/m², which is greater than the 97th percentile for boys his age. At first, Darryl's mother wasn't too concerned. She, too, has always been very heavy. At 5'5" tall, Glenda weighs well over 200 lbs. Her daughter, Taja, is also, according to Glenda, "a little chunky." Darryl also dismissed the issue of his weight. In his words, "I'm not that big. There's plenty of kids bigger than me at school."

Glenda's attitude began to change after she visited her family doctor for a checkup. Just thirty years old, Glenda's doctor found that she was not only obese but also had high cholesterol and high blood pressure. With a stern warning, he urged Glenda and her family to pursue a healthier lifestyle. Glenda's father died of a heart attack at age thirty-nine. Gradually this fact and her doctor's advice persuaded Glenda to commit to changes that would benefit her family.

Darryl eats whatever is available at home and at school. He is actually very physically active. He plays baseball in the summer and basketball with his friends almost every day indoors after school during the colder months. Darryl has a television in his bedroom that he likes to watch for an hour or two before going to bed. He also spends a lot of time watching television on weekends. Glenda takes her kids to fast-food restaurants roughly once per week for dinner. The usual family meals are frozen dinners and pizzas. Glenda and her kids always eat dinner together. Darryl's biggest problem is his gargantuan thirst for soft drinks. A convenience store near his school offers "any size" of fountain drink for eighty-nine cents. Darryl always chooses a huge, 32-ounce drink of root beer. His mom keeps the refrigerator well stocked with 2-liter plastic bottles of regular root beer and cola. In addition to an almost daily 32-ounce fountain drink, Darryl goes through nearly an entire 2-liter bottle of root beer at home.

A Question for You to Consider

Glenda is a busy single mother with limited resources. What one or two simple changes could she make to help her entire family achieve a healthier weight?

ON HIS WAY TO A HEALTHIER WEIGHT

Glenda began initiating changes by establishing two very ambitious behavioral goals: making her home "TV free" and eliminating soft drinks from the family's diet. Glenda has always realized that Darryl hasn't lived up to his academic potential. She felt that getting rid of TV would encourage him to read and do better in school. She rarely watches TV. A week of monitoring revealed that Darryl was watching an average of three hours of TV daily. The family does not have a computer or video game console at home. Glenda sold both of the family's TVs to a secondhand store for $25 each. The first couple of weeks were painful. Darryl felt like his entire bedtime routine had been disrupted. Glenda bought him some comic books, and gradually Darryl made reading comics part of his bedtime routine. Taja made more of a fuss. She was in the habit of watching TV after school. Glenda encouraged her to listen to the radio or read. Instead, Taja has been going over to a friend's home to watch TV in the evenings.

Glenda carefully measured how much soft drink Darryl consumed at home over the course of a week and asked him to tell her when he purchased fountain drinks, either at school or from a convenience store. She estimated that her son was consuming roughly 2½ liters of regular soft drinks a day—the equivalent of a staggering 1,200 calories. Glenda then immediately replaced all soft drinks at home with refrigerated, ordinary tap water. Darryl still buys large servings of soda about three times per week and on occasion has soft drinks at the homes of friends. Glenda is trying to encourage him to get smaller serving sizes.

Darryl's school performance did not improve substantially within six months of the changes described above. His teacher did remark, however, on a recent report card that Darryl seems "less fidgety than usual." Glenda has noticed the same thing. Darryl's interest in comic books has blossomed. He no longer misses TV. Six months after the family made a commitment to pursue a healthier lifestyle, Darryl has lost eight pounds, which is a more significant change than you might think at first, given that he is still growing. He is drinking roughly a third of the amount of soft drink he drank before.

PAULA'S STORY

Paula is the darling of the Martinez family. Paula's mother, Stella, and father, Rodrigo, confess that they and their extended family have spoiled their youngest daughter with affection and junk food. Paula is six years old. She lives in a lower-middle-class neighborhood in Hayward, California, with her parents and ten-year-old sister, Lucia. Rodrigo is a diesel mechanic who works in a truck repair center in San Leandro. Stella stays at home and looks after both her children and her cousin's four-year-old son.

Stella and Rodrigo first became concerned about Paula's weight when Paula's pediatrician told them that their daughter was gaining weight much too fast and was heavier than 95% of girls her age. Stella was particularly upset about this. She blamed herself. She told Paula's doctor, "I know it's my fault. After school, she bugs me for chips, pop, and stuff like that. I usually give in." Stella and Lucia are both fit and trim. Rodrigo is very heavyset and is now trying to cut back on fast food. There is a strong family history of type 2 diabetes on both sides of the Martinez family.

According to Stella, Paula has a voracious appetite for a little girl. The family is a frequent customer of fast-food restaurants, of which there are many in the neighborhood. Paula will usually demand and eat an entire adult meal, usually consisting of a burger, fries, and a

regular soft drink. At home, she asks for and receives generous por-
tions at suppertime. When dining at home, Paula has her choice of one
of several drinks with dinner. She usually chooses cola or orange
soda. Over the past year, Stella has tried to limit Paula's intake of
sweets. She makes sure, for example, that Paula has "only one cookie
a day." Unfortunately, Paula's grandparents live near the family and
visit frequently, bringing with them lots of candy and other sweets to
indulge their granddaughter. Paula looks forward to her grandpar-
ents' visits for this reason and eats these "special treats" until her
"tummy hurts."

Paula is not yet involved in any organized sports, but she is quite
active outdoors throughout the year. She enjoys playing outside with
other kids in the neighborhood. Indeed, Lucia is often sent out on mis-
sions to go find her little sister and drag her back home in time for
dinner. The entire family watches TV together in the evening. Paula
doesn't have a television in her bedroom.

Paula is 4 feet tall and weighs 83 lbs. Her BMI is 25.4 kg/m^2,
which is greater than the 97th percentile for six-year-old girls.

Questions for You to Consider

Paula is a member of a Mexican American family with a strong history of type 2 diabetes. In addition to type 2 diabetes, for which conditions is Paula at increased risk because of her weight?

What recommendations would you make to the Martinez family to
help Paula achieve a healthier weight?

ON HER WAY TO A HEALTHIER WEIGHT

Mexican Americans, like some other ethnic groups, do indeed have an
increased risk for type 2 diabetes.[3] As discussed in chapter 2, type 2
diabetes is the end result of a process that begins with insulin resis-
tance. Obesity promotes insulin resistance. Paula's family history and

ethnicity puts her at risk not only for type 2 diabetes but also for other components of the insulin resistance syndrome including high blood pressure, high cholesterol, and heart disease.

Paula's pediatrician explained the seriousness of obesity to Stella and Rodrigo. The couple identified two principal culprits: the tendency for extended family members to give in to Paula's frequent requests for unhealthy foods and the family's reliance on local fast-food restaurants for meals. Paula's parents' most important goals were reducing Paula's intake of sweets and eliminating her intake of soft drinks. A week of careful monitoring revealed that Paula drinks roughly 300 calories in regular soft drinks per day. They did not feel that they could give up fast-food restaurants since they are so convenient and the couple didn't feel they had the time to cook meals. Instead, Stella and Rodrigo decided to make smarter choices in fast-food restaurants such as salads with low-calorie dressing instead of burgers. Paula loves french fries with ketchup. Stella decided that she had to get used to fresh carrots in their place. Regular soft drinks from fast-food restaurants were to be replaced by ordinary water (generally available free of charge).

Stella told her parents (Paula's grandparents) not to bring treats with them to the family home. Instead, Stella decided to purchase these items and offer them on occasion like any other food alongside healthier snacks. No restrictions would be placed on the quantities. Stella and Rodrigo also decided to make their home "soft drink free." Soft drinks were replaced with low-fat milk.

Rodrigo is a soccer enthusiast. Though both his daughters are fairly physically active, he decided to take them both out to a local park a couple of times a week to teach them basic skills. He felt this would also help him keep his weight under control.

Six months after putting in place a plan to help Paula achieve a healthier weight, she has grown an inch and lost six pounds. She remains the darling of the Martinez family, only a bit slimmer.

Afterword

I am writing this conclusion to my book after a long day of caring for overweight and obese children at the Weight Management Center at Children's Hospital of Pittsburgh. It was a fairly typical busy day. It began with an encounter with a couple of brothers, ages 11 and 12, brought by their father, himself obese, and who had suffered a heart attack last year. After my detailed evaluation, he stopped me in a corridor and told me emphatically, "I just don't want my boys to wind up like me." I saw a seventeen-year-old girl today who told me she desperately wanted to be thin and had tried every diet known to mankind without success. Her friends were all skinny and popular. It took a long time to convince her that the best reason to lose weight is to live a longer, healthier life. My most interesting and challenging patient came in at the end of the day, around 5:30 PM.

Katie (not her real name) is a pretty six-year-old girl who is significantly overweight. I saw her three months ago. After a detailed medical evaluation, she met with a nutritionist who provided her with specific eating and physical activity goals, and identified behaviors that Katie must change in order to lose weight safely. The nutritionist, Katie's parents, and even Katie signed a "contract" which stated that the family would do their best to meet the goals within the next three months. When she returned today, Katie had gained ten pounds and had grown less than half an inch and none of her behaviors had changed. The encounter with Katie and her family began with a long moment of frustration. Her parents were frustrated because they felt they had made their best effort and still failed. I was frustrated because, unlike Katie, all the other children who returned for follow-up appointments today were meeting their goals and losing weight. Katie was frustrated because her parents seemed perpetually unhappy with her. I was frank with Katie's mother and father.

"Katie has gained weight. It sounds like you really haven't changed anything at home."

Katie's father responded after glancing at Katie with exasperation.

"Well, doc, we've tried our hardest. Katie's grandparents live down the street. She'll have dinner at our place and then head over there, and they will feed her all sorts of junk. Katie also sneaks junk food from the kitchen when we're not looking. We've tried to get her to stop drinking soda, but she makes such a big fuss about it sometimes. She also gets pop at school. I don't know what we can do. We feel *helpless.*"

It is hard to deal with such excuses. I could have said, "Can't you convince Katie's grandparents to stop giving her unhealthy snacks?" I was certain that that response would have been met with more excuses. The underlying problem was not the family's desire to help their daughter but that the family did not feel *empowered* to make the necessary changes. To them, Katie's weight had taken on a life of its own, something out of control against which they had battled frequently and lost.

Much of the task of an obesity specialist is to convince patients that something is both important and achievable. Most families recognize that obesity has important consequences. That is why they've made the effort to come to my center. Convincing a family that adopting the behaviors needed to reach a healthy weight is an achievable goal that requires empowering them not only with the required tools but also with the confidence and determination to succeed. This is the last ingredient that you'll need to help your child achieve or maintain a healthy weight. Helping your child achieve a healthy weight is not easy. It takes knowledge of the consequences and causes of obesity as well as "what works" and how to make "what works" an integral part of your family's life. I've provided you with all this information with an added touch of inspiration in the form of stories of children who have met their weight-loss goals. None of this will have any effect unless you realize, unlike Katie's parents, that *no loving parent is helpless*. The fact that you bought and read this book is already a sign of your determination to succeed. Now put the book down and start your child on his way to a fit, trim, and happy future!

Goutham Rao, MD
Pittsburgh, Pennsylvania

Notes

CHAPTER ONE: HOW BAD IS THE PROBLEM?

1. International Food Information Council. Trends in Obesity-Related Media Coverage. Available from: http://www.ific.org/research/obesitytrends .cfm. Accessed October 13, 2004.

2. Centers for Disease Control. BMI for Children and Teens. Available from: http://www.cdc.gov/nccdphp/dnpa/bmi/bmi-for-age.htm. Accessed October 13, 2004.

3. Hedley AA, Ogden CL, Johnson CL, Carroll MD, Curtin LR, Flegal KM. Prevalence of Overweight and Obesity among US Children, Adolescents, and Adults, 1999–2002. *Journal of the American Medical Association.* 2004;291:2847–2850.

4. Ogden CL, Flegal KM, Carroll MD, Johnson CL. Prevalence and Trends in Overweight among US Children and Adolescents, 1999–2000. *Journal of the American Medical Association.* 2002;288:1728–1732.

5. Hedley AA, et al. Prevalence of Overweight and Obesity among US Children, Adolescents, and Adults, 1999–2002.

6. Ibid.

7. Troiano RP, Flegal KM, Kuczmarski RJ, Campbell SM, Johnson CL. Overweight Prevalence and Trends for Children and Adolescents: The National Health and Nutrition Examination Surveys, 1963 to 1991. *Archives of Pediatric Adolescent Medicine.* 1995;149:1085–1091.

8. NIDDK. Statistics Related to Overweight and Obesity. Available from: http://www.niddk.nih.gov/health/nutrit/pubs/statobes.htm#econ. Accessed October 21, 2004.

9. Ibid.

10. Strong JP, Malcom GT, McMahan CA, Tracy RE, Newman WP 3rd, Herderick EE, Cornhill JF. Prevalence and Extent of Atherosclerosis in Adolescents and Young Adults: Implications for Prevention from the Pathobiological Determinants of Atherosclerosis in Youth Study. *Journal of the American Medical Association.* 1999;281(8):727–735.

11. Reaven GM. Banting Lecture 1988. Role of Insulin Resistance in Human Disease. *Nutrition.* 1997;13(1):65.

12. Steinberger J, Daniels SR. Obesity, Insulin Resistance, Diabetes and Cardiovascular Risk in Children. *Circulation* 2003;107:1448–1453.

13. Whitaker RC, Wright JA, Pepe MS, Seidel KD, Dietz WH. Predicting Obesity in Young Adulthood from Childhood and Parental Obesity. *New England Journal of Medicine.* 1997;337:869–873.

14. Pinhas-Hamiel O, Dolan LM, Daniels SR, Standiford D, Khonry PR, Zeitler P. Increased Incidence of Non-Insulin-Dependent Diabetes Mellitus among Adolescents. *Journal of Pediatrics.* 1996;128:608–615.

15. Vargas I. Type 2 Diabetes in Children and Adolescents. Available from: http://nydailynews.healthology.com/nydailynews/15458.htm. Accessed October 15, 2004.

16. Strauss RS. Childhood Obesity. *Current Problems in Pediatrics.* 1999; 29:1–29.

17. Stenius-Aarniala B, Poussa T, Kvarnstrom J, Gronlund EL, Ylikahri M, Mustajoki P. Immediate and Long Term Effects of Weight Reduction in Obese People with Asthma: Randomised Controlled Study. *British Medical Journal.* 2000;320:827–832.

18. Ibid.

19. Tantisira KG, Weiss ST. Complex Interactions in Complex Traits: Obesity and Asthma. *Thorax.* 2001;56(Suppl 2):ii64–ii73.

20. Wing YK, Hui SH, Pak WM, Ho CK, Cheung A, Li AM, Fok TF. A Controlled Study of Sleep Related Disordered Breathing in Obese Children. *Archives of Diseases of Children.* 2003;88(12):1043–1047.

21. Blume J. *Blubber.* New York: Simon & Schuster Books for Young Readers; 1974:79–80.

22. Blume J. *Blubber*. Available from: http://www.judyblume.com /blubber.html. Accessed October 19, 2004.

23. Puhl R, Brownell KD. Bias, Discrimination and Obesity. *Obesity Research*. 2001;9:788–805.

24. Wadden TA, Stunkard AJ. Social and Psychological Consequences of Obesity. *Annals of Internal Medicine*. 1985;103:1062–1067.

25. Flanagan SA. Obesity: The Last Bastion of Prejudice. Available from: http://www.obesity-online.com/ifso/lecture_Flanagan.htm. Accessed October 16, 2004.

26. Stradmeijer M, Bosch J, Koops W, Seidell J. Family Functioning and Psychosocial Adjustment in Overweight Youngsters. *International Journal of Eating Disorders*. 2000;27:110–114.

27. Grilo CM, Wilfey DE, Brownell KD, Rodin J. Teasing, Body Image, and Self-Esteem in a Clinical Sample of Obese Women. *Addictive Behaviors*. 1994;19:443–450.

28. Pesa JA, Syre TS, Jones E. Psychosocial Differences Associated with Body Weight among Female Adolescents: The Importance of Body Image. *Journal of Adolescent Health*. 2000;26:330–337.

29. Israel AC, Ivanova MY. Global and Dimensional Self-Esteem in Pre-Adolescent and Early Adolescent Children Who Are Overweight: Age and Gender Differences. *International Journal of Eating Disorders*. 2002; 31:424–449.

30. Zametkin A, Zoon CK, Klein HW, Munson S. Psychiatric Aspects of Child and Adolescent Obesity: A Review of the Past 10 years. *Journal of the American Academy of Child and Adolescent Psychiatry*. 2004;43(2):134–150.

31. Buddeburg-Fisher B, Klaghofer R, Reed V. Associations between Body Weight, Psychiatric Disorders and Body Image in Female Adolescents. *Psychotherapy and Psychosomatics*. 1999;68:325–332.

32. Britz B, Siegfried W, Ziegler A, Lamertz C, Herpertz-Dahlmann BM, Remschmidt H, Wittchen HU, Hebebrand J. Rates of Psychiatric Disorders in a Clinical Study Group of Adolescents with Extreme Obesity and in Obese Adolescents Ascertained via a Population Based Study. *International Journal of Obesity and Related Metabolic Disorders*. 2000;24(12):1707–1714.

33. Stradmeijer M, et al. Family Functioning and Psychosocial Adjustment in Overweight Youngsters.

34. Canning H, Mayer J. Obesity—Its Possible Effect on College Acceptance. *New England Journal of Medicine*. 1966; 275:1172–1174.

35. Crandall CS. Do Heavy-weight Students Have More Difficulty Paying for College? *Personality and Social Psychology Bulletin.* 1991;17:606–611.

36. Klassen ML, Jasper CR, Harris RJ. The Role of Physical Appearance in Managerial Decisions. *Journal of Business Psychology.* 1993; 8:181–898.

37. Pingitoire R, Dugoni R, Tindale S, Spring B. Bias against Overweight Job Applicants in a Simulated Employment Interview. *Journal of Applied Psychology.* 1994;79:909–917.

38. Roehling MV. Weight-based Discrimination in Employment: Psychological and Legal Aspects. *Personnel Psychology.* 1999;52:969–1017.

39. Register CA, Williams DR. Wage Effects of Obesity among Young Workers. *Social Science Quarterly.* 1990;71:130–141.

40. Pagan JA, Davila A. Obesity, Occupational Attainment, and Earnings. *Social Science Quarterly.* 1997;78:756–770.

41. Flanagan SA. Obesity: The Last Bastion of Prejudice.

42. Klein D, Najman J, Kohrman AF, Munro C. Patient Characteristics That Elicit Negative Responses from Family Physicians. *Journal of Family Practice.* 1982;14:881–888.

43. Bagley CR, Conklin DN, Isherwood RT, Pechiulis DR, Watson LA. Attitudes of Nurses toward Obesity and Obese Patients. *Perceptual and Motor Skills.* 1989;68:954.

44. Wiese HJ, Wilson JF, Jones RA, Neises M. Obesity Stigma Reduction in Medical Students. *International Journal of Obesity and Related Metabolic Disorders.* 1992;16:859–868.

45. Adams CH, Smith NJ, Wilbur DC, Grady KE. The Relationship of Obesity to the Frequency of Pelvic Examinations: Do Physician and Patient Attitudes Make a Difference? *Women Health.* 1993;20:45–57.

CHAPTER TWO: "LIQUID CANDY"

1. US Department of Agriculture. Per Capita Consumption of Major Food Commodities: United States, 1991–2000. Cited July 22, 2004. Available from: http://www.nass.usda.gov/ut/Pdf/ab02/130.pdf.

2. Fawkes H. Pork Choc on the Menu in Ukraine. BBC News. June 21, 2004. Available from: http://news.bbc.co.uk/2/hi/europe/3825221.stm.

3. Bellis M. Introduction to Pop: The History of Soft Drinks. About.com. Available from: http://inventors.about.com/library/weekly/aa092399.htm.

4. Bellis M. The History of Coca-Cola. About.com. Available from: http://inventors.about.com/library/inventors/blcocacola.htm.

5. Coca-Cola Stories. Coca-Cola Co. Available from: http://www2.coca-cola .com/heritage/stories/affordable.html.

6. Peterson MF. Liquid Candy: How Soft Drinks Are Harming Americans' Health. Center for Science in the Public Interest. Available from: http://www.cspinet.org/sodapop/liquid_candy.htm.

7. National Soft Drink Association (NSDA). Available from: http://www.nsda.org/softdrinks/History/funfacts.html.

8. Indiana Dairy Council. Soft Drinks in Schools—A Summary of the Policy Statement from the American Academy of Pediatrics, January 2004. Cited July 22, 2004. Available from: http://www.indianadairycouncil .org/dcc_issues_images/dcc_pages_art_for_archive/21_softdrnks_schools.pdf.

9. Peterson MF. Liquid Candy.

10. Lin BH, Ralston K. Competitive Foods: Soft Drinks vs. Milk. US Department of Agriculture. *Food Assistance and Nutrition Research Report.* 2003;34(7).

11. Ludwig DS, Peterson KE, Gortmaker SL. Relation between Consumption of Sugar-Sweetened Drinks and Childhood Obesity: A Prospective, Observational Analysis. *Lancet.* 2001;357(9255):505–508.

12. Mattes RD. Dietary Compensation by Humans for Supplemental Energy Provided as Ethanol or Carbohydrate in Fluids. *Physiology and Behavior.* 1996;59(1):179–187.

13. Hogbin MB, Hess MA. Public Confusion over Food Portions and Servings. *Journal of the American Dietetic Association.* 1999;99(10): 1209–1211.

14. Rao G. Preferred Serving Size of Soft Drinks among Preadolescents. (Unpublished study funded by the American Academy of Family Physicians, 2003.)

15. McConahy KL, Smiciklas-Wright H, Mitchell DC, Picciano MF. Portion Size of Common Foods Predicts Energy Intake among Preschool-Aged Children. *Journal of the American Dietetic Association.* 2004;104(6): 975–979.

16. Truestarhealth.com. Pop Increases Diabetes Risk in Women. Available from: http://www.truestarhealth.com/members/cm_archives03ML4P1A54.html.

17. Chester D, ed. Disparities in Oral Health in America. *The Oral Care Report*. 2000;10(3).

18. American Dental Association. Joint Report of the American Dental Association Council on Access, Prevention, and Interprofessional Relations and Council on Scientific Affairs to the House of Delegates. Response to resolution 73H-2000. October 2001.

19. Larsen MJ, Richards A. Fluoride Is Unable to Reduce Dental Erosion from Soft Drinks. *Carries Research*. 2002;36:75–80.

20. Wyshak G. Teenaged Girls, Carbonated Beverage Consumption, and Bone Fractures. *Archives of Pediatric and Adolescent Medicine*. 2000; 154(6):610–613.

21. McGartland C, Robson PJ, Murray L, Cran G, Savage MJ, Watkins D, Rooney M, Boreham C. Carbonated Soft Drink Consumption and Bone Mineral Density in Adolescence: The Northern Ireland Young Hearts Project. *Journal of Bone and Mineral Research*. 2003;18(9):1563–1569.

22. Hughes JR, Hale KL. Behavioral Effects of Caffeine and Other Methylxanthines on Children. *Experimental Clinical Psychopharmacology*. 1998;6(1):87–95.

23. Savoca MR, Evans CD, Wilson ME, Harshfield GA, Ludwig DA. The Association of Caffeinated Beverages with Blood Pressure in Adolescents. *Archives of Pediatric and Adolescent Medicine*. 2004;158(5):473–477.

24. Cullen KW, Ash DM, Warneke C, de Moor C. Intake of Soft Drinks, Fruit-Flavored Beverages, and Fruits and Vegetables by Children in Grades 4 through 6. *American Journal of Public Health*. 2002;92(9):1475–1478.

25. Strasburger VC. Children and TV Advertising: Nowhere to Run, Nowhere to Hide. *Journal of Developmental and Behavioral Pediatrics*. 2001;22:185–187.

26. Borzekowski DJG, Robinson TN. The 30-second Effect: An Experiment Revealing the Impact of Television Commercials on Food Preferences of Preschoolers. *Journal of the American Dietetic Association*. 2001;101: 42–46.

27. Ibid.

28. Wechsler H, Brener ND, Kuester S, Miller C. Food Service and Foods and Beverages Available at School: Results from the School Health Policies and Programs Study 2000. *Journal of School Health*. 2001; 71(7):313–323.

29. Lin BH, Ralston K. Competitive Foods.

30. Story M, Hayes M, Kalina B. Availability of Foods in High Schools: Is There Cause for Concern? *Journal of the American Diet Association.* 1996;96:123–126.

31. Nestle M. Soft Drink "Pouring Rights": Marketing Empty Calories. *Public Health Reports* 2000;115:308–319.

32. Fullerton J. Mounting Debt. *Education Next.* Winter 2004:11–19.

33. Associated Press. Reading, Writing and Revenue: Cash-Strapped Schools Turn to Marketing Deals. Available from: http:www.cnn.com /2004/EDUCATION/01/15/schools.commercialism.ap.

34. Nestle M. Soft Drink "Pouring Rights."

35. Lin BH, Ralston K. Competitive Foods.

36. Robertson J. Sweetened Drinks and Children's Health—What Do We Know, and What Can We Do? *Diabetes Technology & Therapeutics.* 2003;5(2):201–203.

37. Bushey J. District 11's Coke Problem. *Harper's.* February 1999:26–27.

38. Molnar A. Sponsored Schools and Commercialized Classrooms. Milwaukee, WI: Center for the Analysis of Commercialism in Education;1998.

39. Wyshak G. Teenaged Girls, Carbonated Beverage Consumption, and Bone Fractures.

40. Nestle M. Soft Drink "Pouring Rights."

41. Fox RF. Warning—Advertising May Be Hazardous to Your Health: Ads Pose a Threat to Physical, Emotional, Social, and Cultural Well-Being. *USA Today Magazine*, November 2001. Available from: http://www.findarticles .com/p/articles/mi_m1272/is_2678_130/ai_80533093.

42. Peterson MF. Liquid Candy.

CHAPTER THREE: FAST-FOOD EPIDEMIC

1. Schlosser E. *Fast Food Nation: The Dark Side of the All-American Meal.* New York: Houghton Mifflin;2001.

2. Bowman S, Gortmaker SL, Ebbeling CB, Pereira MA, Ludwig DS. Effects of Fast-Food Consumption on Energy Intake and Diet Quality among Children in a National Household Survey. *Pediatrics.* 2004;113:112–118.

3. Euromonitor International. Gasoline Station Retailing in the United States. Available from: http://www.euromonitor.com/Gasoline_Station_Retailing _in_United_States. Accessed August 9, 2004.

Meatnews.com. Foodservice and Supermarket Nation. Available from: http://www.meatnews.com/mp/northamerican/dsp_particle_mp.cfm?artNum =364. Accessed September 2, 2004.

American Library Association. Number of Libraries in the United States. Available from: http://www.ala.org/Template.cfm?Section=Library_Fact _Sheets&Template=/ContentManagement/ContentDisplay.cfm&Content ID=22687. Accessed August 9, 2004.

4. Guthrie JF, Lin B-H, Frazao E. Role of Food Prepared Away from Home in the American Diet, 1977–78 versus 1994–96: Changes and Consequences. *Journal of Nutrition Education and Behavior*. 2002;34:140–150.

5. French SA, Story M, Neumark-Sztainer D, Fulkerson JA, Hannan P. Fast Food Restaurant Use among Adolescents: Associations with Nutrient Intake, Food Choices and Behavioral and Psychosocial Variables. *International Journal of Obesity*. 2001;25:1823–1833.

6. Findlaw.com. Ashley Pelman versus McDonald's Corp. Available from: http://www.omm.com/omm_distribution/newsletters/client_alert_class _action/pdf/pelmanmcd90403opn.pdf. Accessed August 9, 2004.

7. Netzer CT. *The Complete Book of Food Counts*. New York: Dell Publishing;2003.

8. Bowman S, et al. Effects of Fast-Food Consumption on Energy Intake and Diet Quality among Children in a National Household Survey.

9. Pereira MA, Kartashov AI, Ebbeling CB, et al. Fast Food Meal Frequency and the Incidence of Obesity and Abnormal Glucose Homeostasis in Young Black and White Adults: The CARDIA Study. *Circulation*. 2003; 107:35.

10. Mennella JA, Griffin CE, Beauchamp GK. Flavor Programming during Infancy. *Pediatrics*. 2004;113(4):840–845.

11. Shannon C, Story M, Fulkerson JA, French SA. Factors in the School Cafeteria Influencing Food Choices by High School Students. *Journal of School Health*. 2002;72(6):229–234.

12. Glanz K, Basil M, Maibach E, Goldberg J, Snyder D. Why Americans Eat What They Do: Taste, Nutrition, Cost, Convenience, and Weight Control Concerns as Influences on Food Consumption. *Journal of the American Dietetic Association*. 1998;98(10):1118–1126.

13. Boje D. A Brief History of Ronald and His Battle with Speedee the Clown. Available from: http://peaceaware.com/McD/pages/History_of _Ronal_McDonald_Speedee_Wal_Mart.htm. Accessed August 9, 2004.

14. Strategic Alliance Promoting Healthy Food and Activity Environments. Unhealthy Marketing to Kids. Available from: www.eatbettermovemore.org. Accessed August 25, 2004.

15. Boje D. A Brief History of Ronald and His Battle with Speedee the Clown.

16. Palmer EL, McDowell CN. Program/Commercial Separators in Children's Television Programming. *Journal of Communication*. 1979;29:197–201.

17. John DR. Through the Eyes of a Child: Children's Knowledge and Understanding of Advertising. In: Macklin MC, Carlson L, eds. *Advertising to Children*. Thousand Oaks, CA: Sage;1999:3–26.

18. Robertson TS, Rossiter JR. Children and Commercial Persuasion: An Attribution Theory Analysis. *Journal of Consumer Research*. 1975;1:13–20.

19. Christenson PG. Children's Perceptions of TV Commercials and Products: The Effects of PSAs. *Communication Research*. 1982; 9:421–524.

20. Schlosser E. *Fast Food Nation: The Dark Side of the All-American Meal*:47.

21. Reece BB, Rifon NJ, Rodriguez K. Selling Food to Children: Is Fun Part of a Balanced Breakfast? In: Macklin MC, Carlson L, eds. *Advertising to Children*:189–208.

22. McDonalds.com. McDonald's Celebrates 25 Years of Happy Meals with the Return of Ty Teenie Beanie Babies. Available from: http://www .mcdonalds.com/usa/news/current/conpr_07222004.html. Accessed September 2, 2004.

CHAPTER FOUR: MESMERIZED BY THE SCREEN

1. Strasburger VC. Children, Adolescents and Television. *Pediatric Reviews*. 1992;13:145–151.

2. MediaFamily.org. Fact Sheet. Children and Television. Available from: http://www.mediafamily.org/facts/facts_childandtv_print.shtml. Accessed September 10, 2004.

3. Paik H. The History of Children's Use of Electronic Media. In:

Singer DG, Singer JL, eds. *Handbook of Children and the Media*. Thousand Oaks, CA: Sage;2001:15.

4. Ibid.

5. Comstock G, Scharrer E. The Use of Television and Other Film-Related Media. In: Singer and Singer. *Handbook of Children and the Media*:60.

6. Television facts. Available from: http://www2.localaccess.com /hardebeck/killtv2.htm. Accessed September 10, 2004.

7. Maccoby EE. Television: Its Impact on Schoolchildren. *Public Opinion Quarterly*. 1951;15:421–441.

8. Gantz W, Masland J. Television as a Babysitter. *Journalism Quarterly*. 1986;63(3):530–536.

9. MediaFamily.org. Fact Sheet. Children and Television.

10. Gunter B, McAleer J. *Children and Television*, 2nd ed. London: Routledge;1997:17–28.

11. Johnsson-Smaragdi V. *TV Use and Social Interaction in Adolescence: A Longitudinal Study*. Stockholm: Almqvist and Wiksell International;1983.

12. Gunter B, McAleer J. *Children and Television*.

13. Vandewater EA, Shim M, Caplovitz AG. Linking Obesity and Activity Level with Children's Television and Video Game Use. *Journal of Adolescence*. 2004;27:71–85.

14. Hancox RJ, Milne BJ, Poulton R. Association between Child and Adolescent Television Viewing and Adult Health: A Longitudinal Birth Cohort Study. *Lancet*. 2004;364:257–262.

15. Robinson TN, Killen J. Obesity Prevention for Children and Adolescents. In: Thompson J, Smolak L, eds. *Body Image, Eating Disorders and Obesity in Youth: Assessment, Prevention and Treatment*. Washington, DC: American Psychological Association;2001.

16. Coon K, Goldberg J, Rogers B, Tucker K. Relationships between Use of Television during Meals and Children's Food Consumption Patterns. *Pediatrics*. 2001;107:e7.

17. Stroebele N, de Castro JM. Television Viewing Is Associated with Increased Meal Frequency in Humans. *Appetite*. 2004;42(1):111–113.

18. Owens J, Maxim R, McGuinn M, Nobile C, Msall M, Alario A. Television-Viewing Habits and Sleep Disturbance in School Children. *Pediatrics*. September1999;104(3):e27.

19. Sekine M, Yamagami T, Handa K, Saito T, Nanri S, Kawaminami K,

Tokui N, Yoshida K, Kagamimori S. A Dose-Response Relationship between Short Sleeping Hours and Childhood Obesity: Results of the Toyama Birth Cohort Study. *Child Care Health and Development.* 2002;28(2):163–170.

20. Walberg H, Haertel G. Educational Psychology's First Century. *Journal of Educational Psychology.* 1992;84:6–20.

21. Koolstra C, van der Voort T. Longitudinal Effects of Television on Children's Leisure Time Reading. *Human Communication Research.* 1996;23:4–36.

22. Singer MI, Slovak K, Frierson R, York P. Viewing Preferences, Symptoms of Psychological Trauma, and Violent Behaviors among Children Who Watch Television. *Journal of the American Academy of Child and Adolescent Psychiatry.* 1998;37(10):1041–1048.

23. Gentile DA, Walsh DA. Media-Quotient; National Survey of Family Media Habits, Knowledge, and Attitudes. Minneapolis, MN: National Institute on Media and the Family;1999.

24. Cantor J, Omdahl B. Effects of Fictional Media Depictions of Realistic Threats on Children's Emotional Responses, Expectations, Worries and Liking for Related Activities. *Communication Monographs.* 1991; 58:384–401.

25. Medved M. Hollywood's 3 Big Lies. *Reader's Digest.* October 1995: 155–159.

26. Huston AC, Donnerstein E, Fairchild H, Feshbach ND, Katz PA, Murray JP, Rubinstein EA, Wilcox BL, Zuckerman D. *Big World, Small Screen: The Role of Television in American Society.* Lincoln: University of Nebraska Press;1992.

27. Steinfeld J. Statement in Hearings before Subcommittee on Communications of Committee on Commerce (US Senate, Serial No. 92–52: 25–27). Washington, DC: US Government Printing Office;1972.

28. Bjorkqvist K. *Violent Films, Anxiety, and Aggression.* Helsinki: Finnish Society of Sciences and Letters;1985.

29. Huesmann LR. Psychological Processes Promoting the Relation between Exposure to Media Violence and Aggressive Behavior by the Viewer. *Journal of Social Issues.* 1986;42(3):125–139.

30. Bushman BJ, Huesmann LR. Effects of Televised Violence on Aggression. In: Singer and Singer. *Handbook of Children and the Media:*235.

31. Medialiteracy.com. Available from: http://www1.medialiteracy.com /stats_technology.jsp. Accessed September 12, 2004.

32. Yahoo Finance. Available from: http://biz.yahoo.com/prnews /040819/nyfnse02_1.html. Accessed September 12, 2004.

33. Sciencenews.org. Available from: http://www.sciencenews.org/articles /20000226/fob8.asp. Accessed September 12, 2004.

34. Gentile DA, Lynch PJ, Linder JR, Walsh DA. The Effects of Violent Video Game Habits on Adolescent Hostility, Aggressive Behaviors, and School Performance. *Journal of Adolescence*. 2004;27(1):5–22.

35. Ibid.

36. Ibid.

37. Vandewater EA, Shim M, Caplovitz AG. Linking Obesity and Activity Level with Children's Television and Video Game Use.

CHAPTER FIVE: BODIES NOT IN MOTION

1. Allen N. The Akimel O'otham: Pima People. In: Weinstein L, ed. *Native Peoples of the Southwest: Negotiating Land, Water, and Ethnicities*. Westport, CT: Bergin & Garvey;2001:89–98.

2. Arizona Indians Reclaim Ancient Foods. Available from: http://www.spmesquite.com/articles/ancientfoods.html. Accessed September 21, 2004.

3. Allen N. The Akimel O'otham: Pima People.

4. Bennett PH. Type 2 Diabetes among the Pima Indians of Arizona: An Epidemic Attributable to Environmental Change? *Nutrition Reviews*. 1999;57(5, pt. 2):S51–54.

5. Ibid.

6. CBSnews.com. Why Is America So Fat? Available from: http://www.cbsnews.com/stories/2004/07/12/60II/main628877.shtml. Accessed September 21, 2004.

7. PBS.org. *Frontline*. Available from: http://www.pbs.org/saf/tran-scripts /transcript502.htm#3. Accessed September 20, 2004.

8. DeNoon D. Old-Time Fitness in Old-Order Amish. Available from: http://my.webmd.com/content/article/79/96115.htm?z=1728_00000_1000_n b_05. Accessed September 21, 2004.

9. Ekelund U, Sardinha LB, Anderssen SA, Harro M, Franks PW, Brage S, Cooper AR, Andersen LB, Riddoch C, Froberg K. Associations

between Objectively Assessed Physical Activity and Indicators of Body Fatness in 9- to 10-year-old European Children: A Population-Based Study from 4 Distinct Regions in Europe (the European Youth Heart Study). *American Journal of Clinical Nutrition*. 2004;80(3):584–590.

10. Ara I, Vicente-Rodriguez G, Jimenez-Ramirez J, Dorado C, Serrano-Sanchez JA, Calbet JA. Regular Participation in Sports Is Associated with Enhanced Physical Fitness and Lower Fat Mass in Prepubertal Boys. *International Journal of Obesity and Related Metabolic Disorders*. 2004;28(12):1585–1593.

11. Ribeiro JC, Guerra S, Oliveira J, Teixeira-Pinto A, Twisk JW, Duarte JA, Mota J. Physical Activity and Biological Risk Factors Clustering in Pediatric Population. *Preventive Medicine*. 2004;39(3):596–601.

12. Trevino RP, Yin Z, Hernandez A, Hale DE, Garcia OA, Mobley C. Impact of the Bienestar School-Based Diabetes Mellitus Prevention Program on Fasting Capillary Glucose Levels: A Randomized Controlled Trial. *Archives of Pediatric and Adolescent Medicine*. 2004;158(9):911–917.

13. Rowland TW. The Role of Physical Activity and Fitness in Children in the Prevention of Adult Cardiovascular Disease. *Progress in Pediatric Cardiology*. 2001;12:199–203.

14. Mutrie N, Parfitt G. Physical Activity and Its Link with Mental, Social and Moral Health in Young People. In: Biddle SJH, Cavill N, Sallis JF, eds. *Young and Active? Young People and Health-Enhancing Physical Activity: Evidence and Implications*. London: Health Education Authority;1998:49–68.

15. Petruzzello SJ, Landers DM, Hatfield BD, Kubitz KA, Salazar W. A Meta-Analysis on the Anxiety-Reducing Effects of Acute and Chronic Exercise: Outcomes and Mechanisms. *Sports Medicine*. 1991;11:143–182.

16. MacKelvie KJ, Khan KM, McKay HA. Is There a Critical Period for Bone Response to Weight-Bearing Exercise in Children and Adolescents? A Systematic Review. *British Journal of Sports Medicine*. 2002;36:250–257.

17. Centers for Disease Control. Physical Activity Levels among Children Aged 9–13—United States, 2002. Available from: http://www.cdc.gov/mmwr/preview/mmwrhtml/mm5233a1.htm.

18. Kimm SYS, Glynn NW, Kriska AM, Barton BA, Kronsberg SS, Daniels SR, Crawford PB, Sabry ZI, Liu K. Decline in Physical Activity in Black Girls and White Girls during Adolescence. *New England Journal of Medicine*. 2002;347:709–715.

19. Lindquist CH, Reynolds KD, Goran MI. Sociocultural Determinants of Physical Activity among Children. *Preventive Medicine.* 1999; 29:305–312.

20. SGMA International. U.S. Team Sports: Participation Trends and Potential Development. Available from: http://www.sgma.com/press /2002 /press1027950869-18219.html. Accessed September 22, 2004.

21. DiGiuiseppi C, Roberts I, Li L. Influence of Changing Travel Patterns on Child Death Rates from Injury: Trend Analysis. *British Medical Journal.* 1997;314(7082):710–713.

22. Title IX, Education Amendments of 1972. Available from: http:// www.dol.gov/oasam/regs/statutes/titleix.htm. Accessed September 22, 2004.

23. Heinonen E. Too Much Title IX? Available from: http://www.keeping-tracknewsletter.com/archive/index.php?belllap=48. Accessed September 23, 2004.

24. USA Today.com. Title IX's Impact Measurable, 30 Years Later. Available from: http://www.usatoday.com/news/education/2002-06-24-title-ix .htm. Accessed September 23, 2004.

25. Tofler IR, Knapp PK, Drell MJ. The Achievement by Proxy Spectrum in Youth Sports. *Child and Adolescent Clinics of North America.* 1998;7(4):803–820.

26. PBS.org. Sports rage. Available from: http://www.pbs.org/newshour /extra/features/july-dec00/sports_rage.html. Accessed September 24, 2004.

27. Susanj D, Stewart C. Specialization in Sport. How Early? How Necessary? Available from: http://www.coachesinfo.com/category/becoming _a_better_coach/7/. Accessed September 24, 2004.

28. President's Council on Physical Fitness and Sports. Motivating Kids in Physical Activity. *Research Digest.* 2000;3(11). Available from: http://www.presidentschallenge.org/misc/news_research/research_digests/5 9547a.pdf. Accessed September 21, 2004.

29. Fromel K, Formankova S, Sallis JF. Physical Activity and Sport Preferences of 10- to 14-year-old Children: A 5-year Prospective Study. *Acta Universitatis Palackianae Olomucensis Gymnica.* 2002;32(1):11–16.

30. Klint KA, Weiss MR. Dropping In and Dropping Out: Participation Motives of Current and Former Youth Gymnasts. *Canadian Journal of Applied Sports Sciences.* 1986;11:106–114.

31. Horn TS. Coaches' Feedback and Changes in Children's Perceptions of Their Physical Competence. *Journal of Educational Psychology.* 1985;77:174–186.

32. Centers for Disease Control. Physical Activity Levels among Children Aged 9–13—United States, 2002.

CHAPTER SIX: THE FAMILY MEAL IN THE TWENTY-FIRST CENTURY

1. Story M. Family Mealtime: Impact on Diet Quality. Available from: http://www.sne.org/conference/Family_Mealtime_handout.pdf. Accessed September 30, 2004.

2. Bowers DE. Cooking Trends Echo Changing Roles of Women. Available from: http://www.ers.usda.gov/publications/foodreview/jan2000/frjan2000d.pdf. Accessed September 30, 2004.

3. Doiron R. Will Work for Food? Increasingly, Americans Won't and Don't. Available from: http://www.utne.com/web_special/web_specials_2003-08/articles/10813-1.html. Accessed October 1, 2004.

4. Halperin M. Indestructible Pocket Sandwich Reports for Military Duty as Americans Grab Up New Handheld Gourmet Choices. Available from: http://www.ccdsf.com/trendcornernov02.html. Accessed October 3, 2004.

5. Kirwan AV. *Host and Guest*. London: Bell and Galdy;1864.

6. Ritchie CIA. *Food in Civilization. How History Has Been Affected by Human Tastes*. New York: Beaufort Books;1981:63.

7. *The Economist*. Filling the World's Belly. December 11, 2003.

8. White H, Kokotsaki K. Indian Food in the UK: Personal Values and Changing Patterns of Consumption. *International Journal of Consumer Studies*. 2004;28(3):284–294.

9. Geest PLC. Available from: http://www.geest.co.uk/gst/ourmarkets/. Accessed October 4, 2004.

10. Dunne D, Narasimhan C. The New Appeal of Private Labels. Available from: http://hbswk.hbs.edu/item.jhtml?id=489&t=marketing. Accessed September 29, 2004.

11. Gillman MW, Rifas-Shiman SL, Frazier AL, Rockett HR, Camargo CA Jr, Field AE, Berkey CS, Colditz GA. Family Dinner and Diet Quality among Older Children and Adolescents. *Archives of Family Medicine*. 2000;9(3):235–240.

12. Gillespie AH, Achterberg CL. Comparison of Family Interaction

Patterns Related to Food and Nutrition. *Journal of the American Dietetic Association.* 1989;89:509–512.

13. Eisenberg ME, Olson RE, Neumark-Sztainer D, Story M, Bearinger LH. Correlations between Family Meals and Psychosocial Well-Being among Adolescents. *Archives of Pediatric and Adolescent Medicine.* 2004;158(8):792–796.

14. Birch LL, Johnson SL, Jones MB, Peters JC. Effects of a Nonenergy Fat Substitute on Children's Energy and Macronutrient Intake. *American Journal of Clinical Nutrition.* 1993;58(3):326–333.

15. Birch LL, Davison KK. Family Environmental Factors Influencing the Developing Behavioral Controls of Food Intake and Childhood Overweight. *Pediatric Clinics of North America.* 2001;48(4):893–907.

16. Birch L, McPhee L, Shoba B, et al. "Clean Your Plate": Effects of Child Feeding Practices on the Development of Intake Regulation. *Learning and Motivation* 1987;18:301–317.

17. Birch LL, Zimmerman S, Hind H. The Influence of Social Affective Context on Preschool Children's Food Preferences. *Child Development.* 1980;51:856–861.

18. Stanek K, Abbott D, Cramer S. Diet Quality and the Eating Environment of Preschool Children. *Journal of the American Dietetic Association.* 1990;90:1582–1584.

19. Fisher JO, Birch LL. Restricting Access to Palatable Foods Affects Children's Behavioral Response, Food Selection, and Intake. *American Journal of Clinical Nutrition.* 1999;69:1264–1272.

20. Fisher JO, Birch LL. Restricting Access to Foods and Children's Eating. *Appetite.* 1999;32:405–419.

21. Birch LL, Fisher JO. Development of Eating Behaviours among Children and Adolescents. *Pediatrics.* 1998;101:539–549.

22. Anorexia Nervosa and Related Eating Disorders, Inc. (ANRED). Available from: http://www.anred.com/causes.html. Accessed October 4, 2004.

CHAPTER SEVEN: THE TRUTH ABOUT DIETS, PROGRAMS, AND OTHER PRODUCTS

1. Dietandbody.com. Available from: http://dietandbody.com/save .html. Accessed October 31, 2004.

2. Cancercoalition.org. Available from: http://www.cancercoalition .org/faq.html. Accessed October 31, 2004.

3. Cleland RL, Gross WC, Koss LD, Daynard M, Muoio KM. *Weight-loss Advertising: An Analysis of Current Trends*. Washington, DC: Federal Trade Commission;2002.

4. Federal Trade Commission. Available from: http://www.ftc.gov/bcp /conline/edcams/redflag/. Accessed October 31, 2004.

5. FTC Moves to Settle Weight-Loss Patch Claims. Available from: http://southflorida.bizjournals.com/southflorida/stories/2004/03/15/daily43 .html. Accessed November 1, 2004.

6. Justin Leonard's Fitness Infomercial Review. Available from: http://www.fitnessinfomercialreview.com/peel_away_the_pounds.htm. Accessed November 1, 2004.

7. FTC Moves to Settle Weight-Loss Patch Claims.

8. Asontv.com. Available from: http://www.asontv.com/products /1037297513.html. Accessed November 3, 2004.

9. Weightwatchers.com. Available from: http://www.weightwatchers .com/about/prs/wwi_template.aspx?GCMSID=1003161. Accessed October 31, 2004.

10. Weight-control Information Network. Available from: http://win .niddk.nih.gov/publications/choosing.htm. Accessed November 1, 2004.

11. Consumers Union. Available from: http://www.consumersunion .org/products/diet502.htm. Accessed October 27, 2004.

12. Disappointing Diets for Children. Available from: http://my .webmd.com/content/Article/83/97667.htm. Accessed October 20, 2004.

13. Moynihan R. Evaluating Health Services: A Reporter Covers the Science of Research Synthesis. Available from: http://www.milbank.org /reports/2004Moynihan/040330Moynihan.html. Accessed November 5, 2004.

14. Ayyad C, Anderson T. Long-Term Efficacy of Dietary Treatment of Obesity: A Systematic Review of Studies Published between 1931 and 1999. *Obesity Reviews*. 2000;1:113–119.

15. Ibid.

16. Summerbell CD, Ashton V, Campbell KJ, Edmunds L, Kelly S, Waters E. Interventions for Treating Obesity in Children. *Cochrane Database of Systematic Reviews*. 2004(3):CD001872.

17. Ibid.

CHAPTER EIGHT: THE SCIENCE OF CHANGING BEHAVIOR AND ITS ROLE IN WEIGHT CONTROL

1. Cohen S. Putting Out the Smoke. Available from: http://www.med.wayne.edu/Wayne%20Medicine/wm2000/puttingout.htm. Accessed November 18, 2004.

2. A Science Odyssey: People and Discoveries. BF Skinner. Available from: http://www.pbs.org/wgbh/aso/databank/entries/bhskin.html. Accessed November 18, 2004.

3. Baranowski T, Cullen KW, Nicklas T, Thompson D, Baranowski J. Are Current Health Behavioral Change Models Helpful in Guiding Prevention of Weight Gain Efforts? *Obesity Research*. 2003;11:23S–43S.

4. Ibid.

5. Contento I, Balch GI, Bronner YL, et al. The Effectiveness of Nutrition Education and Implications for Nutrition Education Policy, Programs, and Research: A Review of Research. *Journal of Nutrition Education*. 1995;27:277–418.

6. Baranowski T, Cullen KW, Nicklas T, Thompson D, Baranowski J. Are Current Health Behavioral Change Models Helpful in Guiding Prevention of Weight Gain Efforts?

7. Ibid.

8. Ibid.

9. Bandura A. Social Cognitive Theory: An Agentic Perspective. *Annual Review of Psychology*. 2001;52:1–26.

10. Wing RR. Behavioral Approaches to the Treatment of Obesity. In: Bray GA, Bouchard C, eds. *Handbook of Obesity: Clinical Applications*. 2nd ed. New York: Marcel-Dekker;2004:147–167.

11. Ibid.

12. Black DR, Gleser LJ, Kooyers KJ. A Meta-Analytic Evaluation of Couples Weight-Loss Programs. *Health Psychology*.1990;9:330–347.

13. Wing RR, Jeffery RW. Benefits of Recruiting Participants with Friends and Increasing Social Support for Weight Loss Maintenance. *Journal of Consulting and Clinical Psychology.* 1999;67:132–138.

CHAPTER NINE: A RATIONAL APPROACH TO ACHIEVING OR MAINTAINING A HEALTHY WEIGHT

1. Rockett RH, Berkey CS, Colditz GA. Evaluation of Dietary Assessment Instruments in Adolescents. *Current Opinion Clinical Nutrition and Metabolic Care.* 2003;6:557–562.

2. Perry CL, Sellers DE, Johnson C, Pedersen S, Bachman KJ, Parcel GS, Stone EJ, Luepker RV, Wu M, Nader PR, Cook K. The Child and Adolescent Trial for Cardiovascular Health (CATCH): Intervention, Implementation, and Feasibility for Elementary Schools in the United States. *Health Education and Behavior.* 1997;24(6):716–735.

3. American Obesity Association. Available from: http://www.obesity.org /subs/childhood/prevention.shtml. Accessed November 25, 2004.

4. American Academy of Pediatrics. AAP Discourages Television for Very Young Children. Available from: http://www.aap.org/advocacy /archives/augdis.htm. Accessed November 25, 2004. American Academy of Pediatrics. Television and the Family. Available from: http://www.aap.org /family/tv1.htm. Accessed November 25, 2004.

5. Centers for Disease Control. Are There Special Recommendations for Young People? Available from: http://www.cdc.gov/nccdphp/dnpa/physical /recommendations/young.htm. Accessed November 26, 2004.

6. Centers for Disease Control. General Physical Activities Defined by Level of Intensity. Available from: http://www.cdc.gov/nccdphp/dnpa /physical/pdf/PA_Intensity_table_2_1.pdf. Accessed November 26, 2004.

7. James J, Thomas P, Cavan D, Kerr D. Preventing Childhood Obesity by Reducing Consumption of Carbonated Drinks: A Cluster Randomized Controlled Trial. *British Medical Journal.* 2004;328:1237.

8. Pennsylvania WIC Program. Choosing Fast Foods Wisely. http://www.nal.usda.gov/wicworks/Sharing_Center/PA/Child_Obesity_part5 .pdf. Accessed November 28, 2004.

9. TV Turnoff Network. Available from: http://www.tvturnoff.org. Accessed November 28, 2004.

10. Brock B. TV Free Families: Are They Lola Granolas, Normal Joes or High and Holy Snots? Available from: http:// www.tvturnoff .org/brock1.htm. Accessed November 28, 2004.

11. Shape Up America. 10,000 Steps Program. Available from: http:// www.shapeup.org/10000steps.html. Accessed November 28, 2004.

12. Shapeup.org. Tips for Everyday Workouts. Available from: http:// www.shapeup.org/publications/fitting.fitness.in/noframes/workday.htm. Accessed November 28, 2004.

13. Nissenberg SK, Bogle ML, Wright AC. *Quick Meals for Healthy Kids and Busy Parents: Wholesome Family Recipes in 30 Minutes or Less from Three Leading Child Nutrition Experts.* New York: John Wiley & Sons;1995.

CHAPTER TEN: ADVOCACY FOR A HEALTHIER "BUILT ENVIRONMENT"

1. News4Colorado.com. Rail Campaign Anticipated to Cost $3 Million. Available from: http://news4colorado.com/campaign2004/local_story _159123053.html. Accessed December 7, 2004.

2. American Community Survey. Ranking Tables 2002. Available from: http://www.census.gov/acs/www/Products/Ranking/2002/R04T050.htm. Accessed December 7, 2004.

3. America 2004. The Democratic Convention. Available from: http://www.dems2004.org. Accessed December 7, 2004.

4. Ibid.

5. Roberts J. Mississippi State Sues Tobacco Companies. *British Medical Journal.* 1994;308:1455.

6. Moore S. The Profligate President: A Midterm Review of George Bush's Fiscal Policy Performance. Available from: http://www.cato .org/pubs/pas/pa-147.html. Accessed December 7, 2004.

7. Schlosser E. *Fast Food Nation. The Dark Side of the All-American Meal.* New York: HarperCollins;2002:102.

8. Ibid.

9. Humpel N, Owen N, Leslie E. Environmental Factors Associated with Adults' Participation in Physical Activity: A Review. *American Journal of Preventive Medicine.* 2002;22(3):88–99.

10. Sallis JF, Prochaska JJ, Taylor WC. A Review of Correlates of Physical Activity of Children and Adolescents. *Medicine and Science in Sports and Exercise.* 2000;32(5):963–975.

11. Saelens BE, Sallis JF, Black JB, Chen D. Neighborhood-Based Differences in Physical Activity: An Environment Scale Evaluation. *American Journal of Public Health.* 2003;93(9):1552–1558.

12. Painter K. Street Lighting, Crime, and Fear of Crime: A Summary of Research. In: Bennett T, ed. *Preventing Crime and Disorder, Targeting Strategies and Responsibilities.* Cambridge, UK: Cambridge Cropwood Series;1996.

13. Macbeth AG. Bicycle Lanes in Toronto. *ITE Journal.* 1999;38–46.

14. Eubanks-Ahrens, B. A Closer Look at the Users of Woonerven. In: Vernez Moudon A, ed. *Public Streets for Public Use.* New York: Columbia University Press;1991:63–79.

15. Centers for Disease Control. Physical Activity Levels among Children Aged 9–13 years—United States 2002. Available from: http://www.cdc.gov/mmwr/preview/mmwrhtml/mm5233a1.htm. Accessed December 11, 2004.

16. Wechsler H, Basch CE, Zybert P, Lantigua R, Shea S. The Availability of Low-Fat Milk in an Inner-City Latino Community: Implications for Nutrition Education. *American Journal of Public Health.* 1995;85(12):1690–1692.

17. Institute of Medicine. Local Communities. In: Preventing Childhood Obesity: Health in the Balance. Available from: http://www.iom.edu/report.asp?id=22596. Accessed December 9, 2004.

18. Bridges4kids.org. Senate Votes to Move the Fizz Off-Campus. Available from: http://www.bridges4kids.org/articles/6-03/SacBee5-30-03.html. Accessed December 10, 2004.

19. Robertson J, Walter CG. What It Took to Ban Soft Drinks in the LAUSD. Available from: http://www.greenearthinstitute.org/nutrition/Documents/LAUSD_Soda_Ban_1102.pdf. Accessed December 10, 2004.

20. Ibid.

21. Parents Advocating School Accountability. Available from: http://www.pasasf.org. Accessed December 10, 2004.

22. American Academy of Pediatrics. AAP Says Soft Drinks in Schools Should Be Restricted. Available from: http://www.aap.org/advocacy/releases/jansoftdrinks.htm. Accessed December 10, 2004.

23. Cox W, Love J. American Highway Users Alliance: A Tribute to the Dwight D. Eisenhower System of Interstate & Defense Highways. Available

from: http://www.publicpurpose.com/freeway1.htm. Accessed December 12, 2004.

24. Friedman MS, Powell KE, Hutwagner L, Graham LM, Teague WG. Impact of Changes in Transportation and Commuting Behaviors during the 1996 Summer Olympic Games in Atlanta on Air Quality and Childhood Asthma. *Journal of the American Medical Association.* 2001;285 (7):897–905.

25. The *Detroit News.* Sprawling Suburbs May Fuel Obesity. Available from: http://www.detnews.com/2003/health/0308/29/health-256878.htm. Accessed December 12, 2004.

26. WalkbikeNashville.org. Make Biking, Walking to School Safe, CDC Urges. Available from: http://www.walkbikenashville.org/Documents /Cdc.htm. Accessed December 12, 2004.

27. National Center for Bicycling and Walking. Safe Routes to School: Getting Started; Organizing and Advocating for Change. Available from: http://www.bikewalk.org/safe_routes_to_school/SR2S_getting_started.htm. Accessed December 12, 2004.

28. Ibid.

29. Ibid.

CHAPTER ELEVEN: A GLIMPSE OF THE FUTURE

1. Infoplease.com. Available from: http://www.infoplease.com/ce6/ent /A0819929.html. Accessed December 16, 2004.

2. Lemonick MD. Time.com. Visions of the 21st Century: Will We Keep Getting Fatter? Available from: http://www.time.com/time/reports /v21/health/fat_mag.html. Accessed December 16, 2004.

3. Culture Change. Taken for a Ride. Available from: http://www.culture change.org/issue10/taken-for-a-ride.htm. Accessed December 16, 2004.

4. Chen DDT. The Science of Smart Growth. *Scientific American.* December 2000:84–91.

5. Geller AL. Smart Growth: A Prescription for Livable Cities. *American Journal of Public Health.* 2003;93(9):1410–1415.

6. Brookings Institution. A Rise in Downtown Living. Available from: http://www.brookings.edu/dybdocroot/es/urban/top21fin.pdf.   Accessed December 16, 2004.

7. Jacobsen MF, Brownell KD. Small Taxes on Soft Drinks and Snack Foods to Promote Health. *American Journal of Public Health.* 2000; 90:854–857.

8. Reger B, Wootan MG, Booth-Butterfield S. Using Mass Media to Promote Healthy Eating: A Community-Based Demonstration Project. *Preventive Medicine.* 1999;29:414–421.

9. Watermelonpunch.com. Available from: http://www.watermelon punch.com/whirl/2003/03/mcdonalds-trying-to-regain-ground.html. Accessed December 19, 2004.

10. Weigle DS. Pharmacological Therapy of Obesity: Past, Present, and Future. *Journal of Clinical Endocrinology and Metabolism.* 2003;88(6): 2462–2469.

11. Ibid.

12. Ibid.

13. Oudiz RJ. Pulmonary Hypertension, Primary. eMedicine.com. Available from: http://www.emedicine.com/MED/topic1962.htm. Accessed December 19, 2004.

14. Weigle DS. Pharmacological Therapy of Obesity: Past, Present, and Future.

15. Ibid.

16. Arterburn DE, Crane PK, Veenstra DL. The Efficacy and Safety of Sibutramine for Weight Loss. *Archives of Internal Medicine.* 2004;164:994–1003.

17. Ibid.

18. McDuffie JR, Calis KA, Uwaifo GI, Sebring NG, Fallon EM, Hubbard VS, Yanovski JA. Three-Month Tolerability of Orlistat in Adolescents with Obesity-Related Comorbid Conditions. *Obesity Research.* 2002;10(7):642–650.

19. Ibid.

20. Ibid.

21. Ibid.

22. About.com. Packard Study to Investigate Diabetes Medicine for Weight Loss in Children. Available from: http://diabetes.about.com/cs/teens anddiabetes/a/blnmetfstudy104.htm. Accessed December 20, 2004.

23. Weigle DS. Pharmacological Therapy of Obesity: Past, Present, and Future.

24. Ibid.

25. Cani PD, Montoya ML, Neyrinck AM, Delzenne NM, Lambert DM.

Potential Modulation of Plasma Ghrelin and Glucagon-like Peptide-1 by Anorexigenic Cannabinoid Compounds, SR141716A (Rimonabant) and Oleoylethanolamide. *British Journal of Nutrition.* 2004;92(5):757–761.

26. Taggart K. Drug Helps Obese Keep Weight Off. MedicalPost.com 2004;40(45). Available from: http://www.medicalpost.com/mpcontent/article .jsp?content=20041128_130203_4140.

27. Tsao A. Has Obesity Met Its Match? BusinessWeek Online. Available from: http://www.businessweek.com/technology/content/apr2004/tc2004048 _9548_tc122.htm. Accessed December 20, 2004.

28. Steinbrook R. Surgery for Severe Obesity. *New England Journal of Medicine.* 2004;350(11):1075–1079.

29. Ibid.

30. Inge TH, Krebs NF, Garcia VF, Skelton JA, Guice KS, Strauss RS, Albanese CT, Brandt ML, Hammer LD, Harmon CM, Kane TD, Klish WJ, Oldham KT, Rudolph CD, Helmrath MA, Donovan E, Daniels SR. Bariatric Surgery for Severely Overweight Adolescents: Concerns and Recommendations. *Pediatrics.* 2004;114(1):217–223.

31. Ibid.

32. Warschburger P, Fromme C, Petermann F, Wojtalla N, Oepen J. Conceptualisation and Evaluation of a Cognitive-Behavioural Training Programme for Children and Adolescents with Obesity. *International Journal of Obesity and Related Metabolic Disorders.* 2001;25(Suppl. 1):S93–S95.

CHAPTER TWELVE: STORIES OF THREE CHILDREN

1. Rao G. *Primary Care Management: Cases and Discussions.* Thousand Oaks, CA: Sage;1999.

2. Rogers C. *On Becoming a Person.* Boston: Houghton-Mifflin;1961:276.

3. Cossrow N, Falkner B. Race/Ethnic Issues in Obesity and Obesity-Related Comorbidities. *Journal of Clinical Endocrinology and Metabolism.* 2004;89(6):2590–2594.

Web Resources

The Internet contains a wealth of excellent resources to help you to help your child achieve or maintain a healthy weight. Rather than overwhelming you with a complete directory of useful Web sites, I've selected a few that complement the recommendations in chapter 9. All provide useful and valid information free of charge.

REDUCING FAST-FOOD CONSUMPTION

Preparing Nutritious Meals at Minimal Cost
http://www.cnpp.usda.gov/FoodPlans/TFP99/food$pdf.PDF

Recipes and Tips for Healthy, Thrifty Meals
http://www.cnpp.usda.gov/Pubs/cookbook/thriftym.pdf

SIMPLE AND HEALTHY RECIPES FOR KIDS

http://kidshealth.org/kid/recipes

HEALTHY CHOICES AT FAST-FOOD RESTAURANTS

Food Database (*provides the caloric and nutritional value of different foods*)
http://www.calorieking.com/foods/

Nutrition at Fast Food Restaurants
http://walking.about.com/od/diet/a/blfastfood.htm

LIMITING TELEVISION AND OTHER MEDIA USE

TV Turnoff Network
http://www.tvturnoff.org

STARTING A WALKING PROGRAM

http://www.thewalkingsite.com/beginner.html
http://www.creatinghealth.psu.edu/osteo/everyone_ex.html

ENCOURAGING FAMILY MEALS

http://www.extension.iastate.edu/Publications/PM1842.pdf
http://kidshealth.org/parent/nutrition_fit/nutrition/habits.html

ENCOURAGING HEALTHY FEEDING PRACTICES

http://www.hersheys.com/nutrition/children.asp
http://www.dshs.state.tx.us/wichd/nut/pdf/fac23-s.pdf

Index

A-B-C model, 140
accelerometer, 89
Accutrim™. See phenyl-
    propanoloamine
acid reflux, 35
advocacy, definition of, 169
African Americans
    barriers to physical activity, 100
    community food environment,
        189–90
    effect of caffeine, 51
    migration of, 187
    obesity among, 29
    physical activity among girls, 92
    self-esteem, 39
AIDS, 29
Alice's Brady Bunch Cookbook
    (Davis, Newcomer, and
    Smolen), 102
All My Children, 72

Allen, Nathan, 84
American Academy of Pediatrics,
    153, 158, 178
American Automobile Association
    (AAA), 180
American Medical Association, 158
American Obesity Association, 153,
    157
Amish, 88–89
amphctamincs, 192
Anderson, T., 128, 129
antecedents, 140
anxiety, 40
Aptos Middle School, 176–77, 179
asteroids, 82
asthma, 13
Atari, 82
atherosclerosis, 31
Atlanta, GA, 187–88
Ayyad, C., 128, 129

Bandura, Albert, 137, 163, 168
bariatric surgery
    for adolescents, 198
    gastric banding, 197
    gastric bypass, 197
    laparoscopic, 197
Bassett, David, 88
behavior modification, 130, 139–43
behavioral learning theory, 135
Belgium, soccer riot, 95
beltways, 168, 171
bicycle paths, 168, 171
Big Mac, 116, 191
bikeability, 182–83
Blount's disease, 36
Blubber (Blume), 37–38
Blume, Judy, 37
body mass index
    and body fatness, 89
    categories in adults, 27
    categories in children, 27–28
    definition, 26
Borzekowski, D., 52
Boston, MA, 181
Boston Market, 57
bottled water, 45, 177
Boulder, CO, 168
Bozo the Clown, 64
Brady Bunch, The, 102–103
Britain
    changing meal patterns, 105–108
    immigration to, 107
    and Indian food, 107
Brownell, Kelly, 190
Buffalo, NY, 205
built environment

definition of, 169
    importance of, 172–74
Burger King, 57, 64
BusinessWeek, 195

caffeine, 51
California, 85, 175
California Gold Rush, 85
Canada, 45, 58, 108, 181
Canadians, 170
cannibinoid receptor, 195
cardiovascular risk factors, 33
Carter, Marlene, 176
CATCH (Child and Adolescent Trial
    for Cardiovascular Health), 150,
    151
causes of obesity, 43
Centers for Disease Control, 27, 92,
    100, 153, 160, 161
Channel One, 54
Chicago, IL, 182
Children's Hospital of Pittsburgh,
    11, 23, 40, 150, 210
chocolate, 46
cholecystokinin, 195
chronic illness, 12, 35
Clarksburg, WV, 190
classical conditioning, 134–35
clinical trials, phases of, 194
clustering of cardiovascular risk fac-
    tors, 90
Coca-Cola, 46–47, 53–54, 191. *See
    also* Coke
Cochrane Collaboration, 127,
    129–30, 199
Cochrane, Archie, 127

cognitive restructuring, 141
Coke, 55
Colombia, soccer team, 95
community food environment,
    173–74
Compagnie de Limonadiers
    (Lemonade Vendors' Com-
    pany), 46
competitive foods, 53
Complete Book of Food Counts
    (Netzer), 62
Congress, 167
Consumer Reports, 124–25
Coolidge Dam, 85
coronary arteries, 33
Cosby Show, The, 102
custard recipe, 106
Custer's Revenge, 82–83

Democratic National Convention,
    170
Denver, CO, 168
depression
    among obese children, 40
    stigma of, 15
Dexatrim™. *See* phenyl-
    propanoloamine
diabetes
    type 1, 32
    type 2, 32–34, 50
diet books, 21
diet drinks, 51–52
dietary recall, 149
dietary record, 149
"Ditch the Fizz," 156
Dr. Pepper, 56
drugs for obesity, 192–97

Dublin, Louis, 26
Duchess of Windsor, 117

economic impact of obesity, 30–31
Eight Is Enough, 102
evidence-based medicine, 18–21

family meals
    evolution of, 101–105, 108–10
    goals for, 154–55
    tips for, 164–66
fast casual restaurants, 57
fast food
    cutting back, 157–58
    definition of, 57
    goals for, 152–53
    and obesity, 61–63
    why children love it, 63–67
Fast Food Nation (Schlosser),
    58–59, 171
fast-food outlets, 60–61
fat burners, 16
Fat Free Pringles, 191
Federal Trade Commission (FTC),
    118–20
feeding practices
    harmful, 110–14
    tips, 165–66
fenfluramine-phentermine, 192
fen-phen. *See* fenfluramine-phenter-
    mine
Field of Dreams, 173
Florida State University School of
    Medicine, 18
Food and Drug Administration
    (FDA), 196
food restriction, 111–14

food-frequency questionnaires, 149
French cooking, 105–106
fry bread, 86
futurism, 185

Generation X, 45
Gila River, 84
Gila River Reservation, 85
goal setting, 139, 147–49
goals for achieving or maintaining a
    healthy weight, 148–49, 151–55
Gregory (pope), 39

H.R. Pufnstuf, 64–65
handheld meals, 105
Hannover, Germany, 173
Happy Meal, 67
Harper's, 54
Harvard Business School, 108
Harvard University, 19, 34
HDL cholesterol, 32
health behavior change models,
    135–39
health belief model, 136–37
Heritage Foundation, 171
home meal replacements, 104, 165
Host and Guest (Kirwan), 105
Huhukam, 84

India, 106
Industrial Revolution, 106
insulin, 31–32, 195
insulin resistance syndrome, 31–33
Intellivision, 82
Internet use among children, 81,
    202–203
Interstate Highway System, 181

intervention for behavior change,
    135–36
irritable bowel syndrome, 117–18

Jacobson, Michael, 47, 190
Jenner, Edward, 186
Joslin, Elliott, 87
juice, 44

Kimm, Sue, 92
Kirwan, A. V., 105
knowledge-attitude behavior model,
    136
Koolstra, C., 79

Lancet, 74
Latinos
    barriers to physical activity, 100
    physical activity among, 93
    preference for whole milk,
        173–74
    self-esteem among girls, 39
Lawson, Nigella, 107, 165
LDL cholesterol, 32
Leave It to Beaver, 102–103
Lemonick, Michael, 186
leptin, 194–95
Lind, James, 126–27
liquid candy, 48
London, UK, 173
Los Angeles, 61, 176
Los Angeles Unified School District
    (LAUSD), 175, 176
low-carb
    diet books, 21
    diets (Atkins), 140
    soft drinks, 191

Maine, 188
marijuana, 195
Matthews, Joseph, 46
McDonald's
  healthier choices, 158, 191
  outlets, 61
  playlands, 66, 67
McDonaldland, 64
McGill University, 19
McLean Deluxe, 191
McMaster University, 18
media coverage of obesity, 24–25, 36
Medicare, 13
Medieval English cooking, 106
Medved, Michael, 80
Mennella, J. A., 63
Meridia™. *See* sibutramine
mesquite bean, 85
metformin, 194
Mexican Americans, 29, 209–10
microwavable meals, 104
Minute Meals, 165
Montreal, QC, 58
Munchkin Bottling Inc., 56

Napa, CA, 60
National Educational Association, 158
National Health and Nutrition
  Examination Survey, 28
National Institutes of Health (NIH),
  194
New England Journal of Medicine,
  92
New York City, 181
New Zealand, 73, 156
norepinephrine, 193

Obama, Barack, 170
Ohio State University, 94
Olestra, 110–11
Oliver, Jamie, 107, 165
operant conditioning, 135
Orlando, FL, 187
orlistat, 193–94
osteoporosis, 51, 91
outcome expectancies, 138

PacMan, 82
paella, 105
Panera Bread Co., 57, 58
Parents Advocating School
  Accountability, 176–77
Paris, France, 19
Pavlov, I., 134–35
peak bone mass, 91
Pedestrian and Bicycle Information
  Center, 183
pedometers, 161
Pennsylvania State University, 112,
  113
Pepsi, 54–55, 191
perceived physical competence,
  96–97, 163
peripheral vascular disease, 33
phenylpropanoloamine, 192
physical activity
  barriers to, 99–100
  fun factor, 97–98
  goals for, 153–54
  habitual, 161
  motivation, 96–99
  patterns among children, 91–93
  social support for, 98–99

tips, 162–64
types of, 91
physical environment, 180–83
Pima Indians
    diabetes among, 87
    history, 84–87
    of Mexico, 87–88
    obesity among, 87
    traditional diet, 84–85
Pittsburgh, PA, 7, 69, 77, 108, 117, 132, 133, 167–68, 181, 189
Pittsburgh International Airport, 58
Portland, OR, 188
pouring rights, 54–55
Power Rangers, 77
prejudice against the obese, 38–42
President's Choice, 108
prevalence of obesity, 28–29
Priestley, Joseph, 46
primary care, 11–12
Primary Care Management: Cases and Discussions (Rao), 200
primary pulmonary hypertension, 192
problem solving, 141–42
psychosocial consequences of obesity, 36–42
PubMed, 22

raising the issue of weight, 14–16
Reading Rainbow, 79
Reaven, Gerald, 31
relapse prevention, 142–43
relaxation
    for weight loss, 130
    progressive muscle relaxation, 199

rimonabant, 195
Roadrunner, 80
Robinson, T., 52
Rodin, Judith, 94
Rogers, Carl, 200
Ronald McDonald, 64–66, 70

Sackett, David, 19
saguaro fruit, 84
San Francisco, 176, 179
sauerbraten, 105
Schlosser, Eric, 58, 171
Scientific Principles of Weight Control, 132–33, 136
Score, Gina, 38
Scott, Willard, 64
scrapple, 88
scurvy, 126–27
sedentary behaviors, 130
self-efficacy, 138, 163
self-monitoring, 140, 149–51
serotonin, 193
Sesame Street, 71, 79
Seven-Up, 56
sibutramine, 193
Simpsons, The, 102
skinfold measurements, 89
Skinner, B. F., 135
sleep-disordered breathing
    apnea, 36
    definition, 35–36
Small Business Administration, 171
smallpox, 186
smart growth, 181, 188
smoking, 48
snoring, 35
social cognitive theory, 137–38

soda. *See* soft drinks
soft drinks
   in baby bottles, 55–56
   and bones, 51
   and compensatory response, 49
   consumption patterns, 47
   and dental caries, 50
   and diabetes, 50
   elimination of, 152, 155–57
   history, 46–47
   labels, 49
   and obesity, 48–49
   in schools, 53–56
   serving sizes, 45
Space Invaders, 82
SpongeBob SquarePants, 78
sports paradox, 93–96
Spurlock, Morgan, 62, 152
stages of change model, 137
Steelers, 95
stimulus-control, 140–41
Stunkard, A. J., 38
Subway, 57
Supersize Me, 58, 62, 64–65, 152, 158
systematic reviews, 125–30, 193

Taken for a Ride, 187
taste preferences of children, 63–64
taxes, on soft drinks and junk food, 190
Teenie Beanie Babies, 67
television
   as babysitter, 70–71
   depiction of family meals, 101–103
   and escapism, 72
   food and drink advertising, 52
   goals for, 153
   and obesity, 73–76
   psychological impact, 79–80
   and radiation, 73
   and reading, 77–79
   reasons for watching, 71–73
   and sleep, 76
   tips for reducing viewing time, 158–60
   viewing time, 69–70
   and violence, 80–81
television advertising perceptions of
   children, 52, 65–67
   and soft drinks, 53
Tesco, 108
theory of reasoned action, 137
Thomas, Dave, 65
thyroid hormone, 192
Time, 186
Title IX, 93–94
tobacco lawsuits, 171
Toronto, ON, 58, 72
transtheoretical model. *See* stages of change model
Tuscany, Italy, 60
TV dinners, 104
TV Turnoff Network, 158–59
TV-free families, 159, 207–208

Ukraine, 46